VITAL VISION
CLEAR EYED SOLUTIONS FOR MIDLIFE AND BEYOND

DR. SAM BERNE

Vital Vision Copyright © 2022 by Sam Berne

All rights reserved.

No part of this book may be reproduced in any form or by any electronic or mechanical means, including information storage and retrieval systems, without written permission from the author, except for the use of brief quotations in a book review.

Colorstone Press
PO Box 458
Tesuque, NM, 87574
1-877-239-3777

CONTENTS

What people are saying about Dr. Berne's work: ... vii
Introduction ... xi

1. **FLOATERS** ... 1
   What are Floaters? ... 1
   When to Visit a Doctor ... 3
   What Factors Lead to Floaters? ... 5
   Will I Need Surgery? ... 11
   Lifestyle Changes To Address Floaters ... 13
   Exercises for Reducing Floaters ... 19

2. **CATARACTS** ... 25
   What are Cataracts? ... 25
   What are the Symptoms? ... 26
   Disease Progression ... 28
   Who is at Risk? ... 29
   What Can I Do About Them? ... 31
   If You Need Surgery ... 40
   Preparing for Surgery ... 43
   What Happens After Surgery? ... 46
   Eye Exercises for Cataract Reversal ... 51

3. **MACULAR DEGENERATION** ... 55
   What Is Macular Degeneration? ... 55
   Types of Macular Degeneration ... 57
   Symptoms and Progression ... 59
   Who is at Risk? ... 61
   When to Visit a Doctor ... 65
   What Can I Do About It? ... 67
   Diet ... 70

Lifestyle Changes	76
Eye Exercises For Macular Degeneration	79

4. MYOPIA & ASTIGMATISM — 83
What are Myopia and Astigmatism?	84
What are the Causes?	86
When to See a Doctor	90
Tips For Your Eye Exam	93
Reduce Your Prescription!	95
Other Recommendations	102
What About Surgery?	110
Eye Exercises for Astigmatism and Myopia	111

5. HYPEROPIA & PRESBYOPIA — 117
What are Hyperopia and Presbyopia?	118
What are the Causes?	120
When to See a Doctor	126
What Can I Do About It?	129
What About Surgery?	137
Eye Exercises for Farsightedness	140

6. STRABISMUS, AMBLYOPIA, AND DIPLOPIA — 145
What are Strabismus, Amblyopia, and Diplopia?	147
What are the Causes?	152
Double Vision	154
When Should I See a Doctor?	159
Standard Treatments	160
The Impact of Vision Therapy	163
Other Treatment Options	166
Eye Exercises for Eye Coordination	169

7. DRUGS AND SURGERY VERSUS HERBS AND AROMATHERAPY — 175
What is the Ocular Microbiome?	175
The Body Heals	180
Essential Oils	181
How to Choose an Essential Oil	189
My Essential Oils Eye Protocol	193

8. NUTRITION TIPS – WHAT TO EAT FOR
   HEALTHY EYES   197
   The State of Diets Today   198
   Gut Health and Vision   202
   Diet, Vision, and Nutrient Absorption   205
   How Diet Affects Your Individual Health   207
   The Rainbow Diet   209
   Healthy Fats   217
   Healthy Drinks   218
   Glossary of Eye-Healthy Super Fruits and
   Veggies   220
   Glossary of Nutrients for Eye Health   224

9. LIGHT, COLOR, AND VIBRATIONAL
   MEDICINE FOR HEALING THE EYES
   AND BODY   233
   What is Light?   234
   Light as Medicine   236
   Color Therapy   244
   My Color Therapy Practice   246
   The Energy Field Hypothesis   251
   Chakras   258

   About the Author   269
   Notes   271
   Acknowledgments   303

WHAT PEOPLE ARE SAYING ABOUT DR. BERNE'S WORK:

Workshop Testimonials

"Dr Berne I think your information from the Neuroplasticity class is awesome!"—Will M

"I can't believe after 3 months of doing your cataract protocol, my cataract went away. It is a miracle! Your cataract class was amazing!" M L

"I had a trauma and PTSD from a car accident. The neuroplasticity protocol reduced my anxiety and panic attacks within a week of taking your course. Your approach is so much better than traditional eye medicine." AL

"I was diagnosed with narrow angle glaucoma and lost part of my visual field. Your class on neuroplasticity has given me more peripheral vision. I can go shopping in a store again. Thank you so much!" JP

"My husband was diagnosed with macular edema and he received regular monthly shots. After taking your course on myopia, he was able to reduce his prescription by 20% and his retina is healing. He now only needs the shot every 3 months. Thank you so much." AS

"Thank you for all the good work you are doing. Since taking your Cataract course, my doctor says I don't need to get surgery right now. Wow, I am thrilled!" BN

"I have been following you on Youtube and I took your class on Reducing Myopia. My goodness my glasses feel too strong, so I went for an exam and my doctor said I reduced my myopia from -3 to -2. What a miracle. Thank you!" YN

"I have suffered computer eye strain for years. After taking your class on Reversing Myopia, I now do the color therapy you taught me and my headaches are completely gone. I am very pleased!" MK

"I found Dr. Berne's, online classes very powerful for releasing tension in the eyes, returning them to greater health. As a developmental trauma specialist, I also recognize how powerful Dr. Berne's work is for addressing deeply held somatic tensions, that may have been limiting life since childhood. I highly recommend his classes" JB Yau, California 2019

INTRODUCTION

I once visited a colleague's office and was shocked to hear the practitioner tell a patient, "At 40 you'll need reading glasses, at 50-bifocals. By 60, you'll need trifocals, and you'll have floaters and a posterior vitreous detachment. At 70 you'll need cataract surgery and probably an iridectomy for glaucoma. At 80, you'll be blind." Even more shocking was the thought that every patient was likely getting a similar message.

The purpose of this book is to counteract that message. Contrary to what this practitioner told their patients, and contrary to what our current healthcare practices dictate, *no matter what your eye condition, you don't have to live with that diagnosis for life.*

A new age of science is upon us where researchers are proving our bodies' inherent ability to heal. Instead of

INTRODUCTION

accepting a diagnosis as a life sentence and smothering it with drugs or cutting it out with surgery at any age, you can unlock your innate regenerative capacity and create new, healthy pathways. Cell regeneration is happening all over the body, all the time. The skin turns over and creates new skin cells every two months. The body is a veritable repository of self-healing mechanisms – even in our eyeballs.

Even those with healthy eyes will benefit from the content of these pages to learn ways to promote bodily self-healing and homeostasis and prevent age-related eye conditions. Through physical eye exercises combined with diet and lifestyle changes, you can preserve and even improve vision at any age. By taking a holistic approach to your eye health, you empower yourself to make your entire body healthier.

ANATOMY OF THE EYE

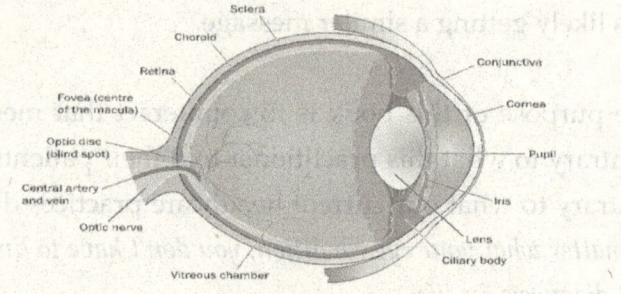

We should start by understanding the anatomy of the eye. Externally, each eyeball has six muscles that control

INTRODUCTION

their movement and are in constant involuntary motion, moving anywhere from 30 to 70 times a second. The eyelid cleans and wets the surface of the eye, and beneath the upper eyelid are glands and ducts that secrete tears.

On the eyeball itself, a thick, tough flexible outer coating called the *sclera* protects its outermost surface, and the clear cornea right beneath it is the part of the eye that first takes in light. The colorful iris expands and contracts to control how much light enters, and the pupil is the opening through which we view light. The light then passes through the lens, which puts it into focus. Behind the cornea, iris, and around the lens is a chamber that contains the aqueous humor, a clear, colorless liquid. The aqueous humor provides nutrients to the transparent parts of the eye.

After the lens, the light then passes through the vitreous body and reaches the light-sensitive retina that lines the back of the eye. Protecting the retina is the choroid, a layer of vascular tissue with a network of microcapillaries responsible for distributing nutrients. This layer is especially important because the retina has one of the highest metabolic needs in our bodies. A healthy retina converts the light into an electrical impulse, which sends it to the visual cortex. From the visual cortex, it gets converted into optical images for the brain's processing and interpretation.

INTRODUCTION

THE EYE-BRAIN-BODY CONNECTION

Only about 10% of the process of seeing is accomplished in the eyeball. The other 90% occurs in the brain, so a healthy brain is essential for sight. When the eyes start developing about 17 days into gestation, the optical vesicles first start to grow directly out from the brain, and every tissue of the eye is the same as our highly absorbent brain tissue. Through this tissue, our eyes connect to our central nervous, endocrine, and fluid systems. As a result, they reflect our biochemical imbalances and even the history of our bodies since birth. This is why an imbalance anywhere in our body invariably affects our eyes.

Our nutrition is intimately connected with eye health. Most of the components of the eye absorb nutrients through the vascular tissue of the choroid and its microcapillaries. Metabolic waste accumulation in the eyes results from a lack of the right nutrients entering into those microcapillaries, further inhibiting nutrient absorption and leaving the eye more susceptible to various conditions.

We're also discovering that our bodily microbiomes are another significant contributor to eye health. You can find these communities of healthy bacteria, viruses, archaea, and eukaryotic microbes in your body, and new research is starting to uncover the mysteries of the microbiome in our eyes. These communities of microbiota protect our bodies against pathogens, support immune system development, and enable the proper metabolism of food into energy. Strengthening our bodily microbiomes can improve cataracts, glaucoma, macular generation, and other problems.

WHERE TRADITIONAL METHODS FAIL

Even as we discover the different ways our bodily systems are integrated with one another, our health care today has become more disconnected and segmented than ever. Gastrointestinal specialists handle the gut, neurobiologists handle the brain, cardiologists handle the heart, and ophthalmologists handle the eyes. But since the healthy functioning of all of these systems depends on one another, this kind of segmented care is becoming increasingly inadequate.

This means our traditional solutions to eye health are only covering up bigger problems. Treating the eyes with prescription lenses actually makes the eyes worse by shutting down the vestibular system and overstimulating the sympathetic nervous system. A lens based on a 20/20 eye chart locks you in a defensive posture. Once you lock your eyes down with prescription lenses, there's very little movement in changing your vision. This is why the first thing I do with a new patient is take off their current lenses and give them a reduced prescription.

INTRODUCTION

Surgery is another traditional option for eye health that does more to cover up the problem than to solve it. When a surgeon operates on your eye, they only change the prescription superficially on the eyeball while its connection with the brain and body remains unchanged. This new programming in the eye conflicts with signals in the brain, creating a mismatch that the brain attempts to resolve. Over time, the eye reverts to its pre-surgical condition.

A HOLISTIC APPROACH

With the dominant belief that prescriptions and surgery are the only options, people can often feel bullied into accepting a certain procedure or treatment method, even if they would prefer another option. If this is you, pause before accepting anything and first seek out a second opinion from a more holistic perspective.

Since so many blood vessels run in and out of the eye, I always recommend getting a physical exam once a year to check your overall blood pressure, heart, and arteries. Functional medicine doctors or naturopaths will run biochemical tests to give you more info on systemic health. You may also choose to see a practitioner of Rolfing, Continuum Movement™, or acupuncture. I particularly recommend the use of vision therapy – a form of physical therapy for the eyes that helps re-educate the eyes, brain, and body to reprogram and develop their ability to function together.

INTRODUCTION

This book describes other methods for improving your eye health, including nutrition, physical therapy, and meditation practices – most of which you can do entirely on your own. These practices are based on a new paradigm that says our environment, lifestyle, and spiritual habits play a more significant role in our health than our genes.

The first step to tapping into this deeper potential of your biological destiny is to embrace your resiliency. Instead of deciding, "My eyes are letting me down," ask yourself, "How am I letting my eyes down?" It's so easy to complain about our eyes: "They hurt. They're dry. Their vision is terrible. Without my glasses, I'm as blind as a bat." While it may be true that your eyes are suffering, instead of trying to blame your eyes for being unhealthy, you should be wondering what it is they need to be healthy. This book will help you answer that question.

DISCLAIMER:

The information in this book is educational and not meant to serve as a substitute for regular visits with your eye doctor. It is, however, meant to guide you towards asking deeper questions about your eye health and how healing your eyes might be linked to healing other systems in your body.

INTRODUCTION

This book includes a combination of right- and left-brain wisdom and may not be for everyone. More traditional readers might question my methods, and my procedure may not help those who doubt its efficacy. But if you are open to a new way of seeing and are willing to join me in exploring new territories, please, keep reading!

CHAPTER 1
FLOATERS

WHAT ARE FLOATERS?

Ever think you see something in the corner of your eye, but when you turn to look, it's gone? While it's easy to believe that you've witnessed some spectral phenomenon, floaters are the more likely culprit. You know the ones – those specks and flecks that float around when you move your eyes, but always manage to escape your line of sight.

You may not have known them by name before, but once you know what to look for, you can easily tell if your eyes have floaters. Try making small eye movements across a white wall, blue sky, or bright screen and focus your attention on any movement that seems to glide through your field of vision. If you see a spot that doesn't exist externally, you likely have floaters.

As many as 60% of us get floaters at some point in our lives. Typically, they are not life-threatening or debilitating, so people may not consider them to be a "big deal." But these innocent specks can become increasingly numerous, taking over more and more of your field of view, impeding your vision, and affecting your everyday life. They also can be a sign of other threats to your eyes.

But the good news is – through a combination of diet and eye exercises, you can get rid of them!

Floaters develop in the vitreous, or *vitreous humor*. This is a colorless, transparent gelatinous sac made up mostly of water and proteins, including collagen. It fills the space between the lens of the eye and the retina. Floaters begin when tiny, undigested proteins clump together and accumulate into visible objects that float in the vitreous. They hover in front of your macula at the center of the retina and cast shadows against it. These shadows appear in your vision as small dark blobs or dots. These may be grey or black and they might take the form of spots, strands, or cobweb-like formations. They may appear directly in the middle of your vision or drift in and out. When you try to focus on them, they may shift along with your eye movement, always escaping direct examination.

WHEN TO VISIT A DOCTOR

In general, the presence of a few floaters on their own does not mean you need to go to the doctor since they can usually exist without harmful effects. But if your floaters become bothersome, it doesn't hurt visit to your eye doctor to bring up your concerns. Having a doctor's confirmation that you have floaters can guide you towards remedies, like those in this chapter, that can improve the eye environment and break up those proteins in the vitreous.

However, you should visit your doctor immediately if many floaters appear at once, or if you start to see flashes along with the floaters. These symptoms could indicate that your vitreous is detaching from either the macula or the retina.

When too much protein accumulates in the vitreous, it can shrink and eventually pull away from the macula, a condition known as *posterior vitreous detachment* (PVD). This may result in blurred vision and visual distortion.

Retinal detachment is a serious condition that can permanently damage your eyesight. When the eye first develops, the vitreous fills in behind it, pressing against and eventually attaching itself to the surface of the retina. As the vitreous dries up and begins to detach, it can tug on the retina and cause a tear, which allows the vitreous to enter the opening. This pressure on the retina can dislodge it from the back of the eye's inner lining. Without this connection intact for receiving vital oxygen and nutrients, the whole eye system suffers.

Visiting a doctor early can confirm any vitreous or retinal detachment and then help you find the source of the floaters so you can treat them. If you've suffered a retinal tear or detachment, a surgeon can reattach the retina and restore visual function. But if you find out about the problem sooner, you can avoid surgery by restoring health to your eyes.

Additionally, if you have diabetes, you should take the presence of any floaters seriously as they may be a sign of *proliferative diabetic retinopathy*. With this eye disease, high blood sugar levels damage the microcapillaries (small blood vessels) in the retina. This can cause bleeding and blood clots, which then leak into the vitreous and lead to floaters. This bleeding can eventually obscure more of your vision or cause retinal detachment.

When you go to your eye doctor about floaters, the more detail you can give, the better. They might ask when you first noticed them, what kind of shape they take and how many you see in your vision. They'll probably ask if you've seen flashes or had any head or eye injuries. During the visual acuity test, they might ask if you see floaters, both at a distance or near. After that, the doctor will put drops in your eyes to dilate your pupils and gives you a dilated retinal exam. With a flashlight, they'll examine the vitreous gel in your eyes for indications of the floating clumps.

It's also possible that what you're seeing in your field of vision aren't true floaters, but objects caused by some other condition. Spasms in blood vessels of the brain can also create jagged waves in both eyes that can last up to 20 minutes. You can also have an ocular migraine or, if you take the heart medication digitalis, it can be a sign of toxicity. If you suspect you have one of these conditions, you should go to a naturopathic or functional medicine physician for treatment.

WHAT FACTORS LEAD TO FLOATERS?

When it comes to eye health, there's no single answer for everybody. The way the eyes function is largely dependent upon the health of all the other systems in the body.

DR. SAM BERNE

This means that disruption in any of those systems can result in these protein clumps in the vitreous. In my experience treating patients with floaters, these are some of the most common reasons they develop.

AGE

As with many eye conditions, floaters become more common with age. As we get older, our bodies require more work to keep them oxygenated and hydrated, which means our eyes dry out and lose nutrients. Without proper hydration, the vitreous is more susceptible to forming clumps. In fact, over 50% of people over the age of 70 will see floaters at any given time.

DIET

Just like the cardiovascular network in the rest of the body, blood vessels in the eyes need nutrients to help eliminate oxidative stress and dehydration. Consuming more antioxidants will help fight off the free radicals that cause oxidative stress and cell damage. (See below for specific dietary tips for reducing your floaters.)

TRAUMA

Trauma to the head shakes up the eyeball and can dislodge the particles that accumulate to make up floaters.

POOR DENTISTRY

About 50% of the material used for dental amalgams, or "silver fillings," used to fill cavities is liquid mercury.[1] Mercury in the body can cause behavioral and neurological disorders, tremors, headaches, mood swings, insomnia, and even blurred vision. Both the mercury amalgams and root canals can influence circulation in and around the eyes and increase oxidative stress, especially in the vitreous, which can result in floaters. I recommend seeking out a biological dentist who treats your mouth from a holistic perspective so that you are reducing toxicity that could be getting absorbed in the eyes.

EMF EXPOSURE

Studies have found that exposure to electromagnetic fields (EMF), things like radio waves, microwaves, and wireless internet, can induce changes in the nerve cells of the central nervous system, even kill them. They also cite EMF as a cause of stress in living creatures.[2] Chronic stress leads to an overall reduction in bodily circulation, which prevents the eyes from absorbing nutrients and creates free radical damage from the metabolic waste. All this build-up further cuts the eye tissue off from necessary nutrients, leaving them susceptible to drying out – thus leading to floaters.

MYOPIA

Floaters might appear in the eyes due to nearsightedness, or myopia. If your vision measures over minus six diopters, this keeps the eye muscles under constant visual stress even if you wear prescription lenses. This can trigger a weakening in the connective tissue. Studies show that the higher myopia, the more likely floaters are to negatively impact your vision[3] and the higher the risk of developing PVD at a younger age.[4] (See Chapter 4, Myopia and Astigmatism, to address your myopia along with your efforts to reduce your floaters.)

CATARACT SURGERY

Many of my patients have reported the appearance of floaters after cataract surgery. If you have cataracts, jumping immediately to a surgical option adds the risk of developing a new eye condition like floaters. Consider instead holistic care that can reduce or eliminate cataracts and promote a healthy eye environment. (See Chapter 2, Cataracts, for more information.)

• • •

MEDICINES

A number of drugs can increase the likelihood of developing floaters. The use of anti-inflammatory steroids, or corticosteroids, can raise eye pressure and lead to floaters. Research shows that patients should notice this pressure diminish within one to four weeks after discontinuing steroid use.[5] The allergy reliever diphenhydramine (Benadryl) and the antianxiety drug alprazolam (Xanax) can both cause floaters because of dehydration of the eye. Elavil, taken for depression, can cause vascular problems in the eye that result in floaters.[6]

CHRONIC INFLAMMATION

If you have hypertension, an auto-immune disease, or other conditions that cause chronic inflammation, this constriction of the blood vessels limits your eye's access to nutrients and hydration.

MOLD

Mold exposure is a significant cause of floaters that has gone largely under the radar. Mold can live anywhere in the body for months or years undetected. We most often associate mold with respiratory problems, but studies also show adverse effects on many bodily systems.[7]

Constant exposure to indoor mold can overwhelm the body, leading to Chronic Inflammatory Response Syndrome (CIRS), symptoms of which include dry, red eyes and blurred vision.[8] These effects are heightened in an estimated 25% of the population who are carriers of the HLA-DR gene,[9] which inhibits the production of antibodies needed to clear mold from the system. You can get a blood test to determine if you carry this gene and the increased risk of side effects it can bring to your eyes.

ALLERGIES

Allergies are caused by the immune system overreacting to an allergen and triggering the release of inflammatory chemicals called histamines. This response usually occurs within two hours of exposure to allergens such as certain foods, drugs, GMO ingredients, smoke, or pollen. Allergic responses reduce the liver's efficiency in cleansing the blood of toxins. The higher the toxic load in the blood, the greater the chance that the vitreous gel will suffer oxidative stress and floaters.

YEAST INFECTION

Also known as a fungal infection, this condition occurs when there is an overgrowth of the yeast that lives in the mouth, throat, gut, and vagina. A yeast infection indicates an acidic body environment, which results in inflammation and poor cellular metabolism. Because of the connection between your eyes and gut health, yeast infections prevent the eye tissues, especially the vitreous gel, from getting the needed nutrients. The vitreous begins to shrink and harden, and the protein from the collagen breaks off and begins floating in the vitreous gel sac.

HEAVY METAL TOXICITIES

These days, we are being inundated with heavy metals like mercury, lead, cadmium, aluminum, and other neurotoxins that rob our eyes and brain of the necessary oxygenation needed to detoxify them. The vitreous is an oxygen-rich area, but when heavy metals and other toxins build up, the collagen breaks down, your vision is blurred and floaters will form. I recommend you get tested to see what your heavy metal baseline is and then start a natural detoxification program by following the dietary recommendations below.

WILL I NEED SURGERY?

When people feel that their large, persistent eye floaters are affecting their quality of life and want them removed immediately, they may want to try surgery. Luckily, available surgical treatments for floaters today are much less invasive than previous risky practices that actually removed parts of the vitreous from the eye along with the floaters. Most doctors now use *laser vitreolysis*, which is usually pain-free and performed right in the ophthalmologist's office.

After applying an anesthetic eye drop, the doctor will use a special lens on your eye and deliver laser energy into the vitreous through a slit lamp to break up the floaters. the doctor will apply anti-inflammatory drops after rinsing your eyes. The process takes no more than half an hour. You may see gas bubbles appearing as small dark spots right after treatment, but these resolve quickly. You may also experience some mild discomfort, redness, or blurry vision, but nothing that should keep you from returning to normal activities.

But would I recommend it? Well, the results aren't so promising. Some patients try laser surgery and end up with more cloudiness in their vision. And while surgery may break up your existing floaters, it does nothing to address what caused them in the first place. That means you'll likely develop new ones unless you make some changes. Instead of resigning yourself to a diagnosis and a medical procedure to address it, you can take control over your eye health by implementing lifestyle practices to heal it yourself.

LIFESTYLE CHANGES TO ADDRESS FLOATERS

Alternatives to surgery are often more successful in the long run because they address underlying causes rather than symptoms alone. Since eye floaters mostly result from a lack of oxygenation and hydration, or some degree of inflammation and metabolic waste build-up, we can broadly address these causes through all systems of the body that interact with eye health. Through the following diet and lifestyle changes, you can break up existing floaters and improve your vitreous environment to prevent the development of new ones.

DIET

To improve your eye health, you need sufficient quantities of collagen, vitamin C, and vitamin A, and you need to rid your body of toxins that build up in the body and cause problems in the vitreous. Both of these can be accomplished with dietary changes.

Collagen, the most abundant protein in the body, serves as the connective tissue in the vitreous. Without enough hydration and nutrients, collagen in the vitreous can weaken and dry out. This is why floaters become more common with age: not only is it more difficult for the body to produce new collagen, but the older we get, the more existing collagen dries out and breaks down. These collagen protein flakes can accumulate in the vitreous and solidify into floaters. In addition to reducing floaters, adding collagen to your diet has a myriad of health benefits. It improves your joint health, metabolism, muscle mass, nails, hair, and teeth. It even slows down the aging process!

Vitamin C supports the maintenance of healthy collagen levels.[1] Especially in combination with hyaluronic acid, it helps to retain tissue moisture throughout the body, including bones, skin, connective tissue, and the eyes. Our bodies produce less hyaluronic acid as we age. Consuming vitamin C along with a hyaluronic acid supplement can improve eye moisture and boost collagen, both needed to help address your floaters.

To produce moisture and stay well-lubricated, your eyes need vitamin A. In a 2019 study on dry eyes, participants noticed better quality tearing after only three days of taking vitamin A supplements.[2] Its antioxidant properties also help to break down free radicals that cause metabolic waste build-up and cut off eye circulation, which can cause floaters.

What foods and supplements should you consume to boost your levels of these important nutrients?

Aloe vera: Best known as a collagen-booster for skin health, when ingested in its pure form or as a supplement, aloe can improve total body collagen, including in the eyes.

Animal products: Bone broth has become a popular collagen booster, but it can also be found in beef, chicken, fish, and eggs.

Veggie broth: Vegans and vegetarians can get into collagen-boosting broth, too. Veggie scraps are full of collagen, so instead of tossing them, store them in a resealable jar in the freezer until you accumulate a quart. Then, slow cook for a few hours with two quarts of water, a half tablespoon of sea salt, and some seaweed until everything softens. Strain and discard the plant parts and enjoy a delicious veggie collagen tea.

Cruciferous Vegetables: Broccoli and brussels sprouts are known for their high antioxidant content that reduces inflammation and oxidative stress.[3] One serving of cooked brussels also provides 53% of your daily recommended intake of vitamin C, and broccoli provides 57%.[4]

Strawberries: One cup of sliced strawberries provides over 100% of your daily recommended vitamin C intake.[5] Studies have shown strawberries to prevent inflammation disorders and oxidative stress,[6] and one study showed a decrease in blood vessel inflammation by 18% over eight weeks of consuming freeze-dried strawberries.[7]

Ginseng: Ginseng's power to eliminate waste products and inhibit vascular endothelial growth factor (VEGF) likely plays a role in reducing the risk for eye diseases.[8] A 2012 study found that ginseng also triggers collagen production and anti-aging effects.[9]

Cilantro: Cilantro contains eye-healthy antioxidants like vitamin A, lutein, zeaxanthin and beta carotene,[10] but is also great for boosting collagen. 100 grams of cilantro contains 30% of your recommended daily vitamin C intake.

Algae: Algae contains important eye nutrients like vitamins A, C, and E, which have demonstrated potential antioxidant, anti-inflammatory, antidiabetic and antihypertensive effects. Studies have also found marine algae extracts to prevent UV-induced oxidative stress and the degradation of skin collagen.[11]

In addition to adding healthy foods to your diet, it's a good idea to go through a liver detox to remove waste products from the body. The exact process for detox will depend on your constitution, current lifestyle, diet, stress levels, and current digestive health – so see your functional medicine specialist for guidance on the best way forward.

A liver detox also impacts the body's *qi*, or life force. According to traditional Chinese medicine (TCM), the body is an interrelated set of systems that work harmoniously, meaning a problem in one part of the body can lead to problems in others. In TCM philosophy, problems arise when something is blocking our *qi*. The liver meridian rules the eyes and the liver *qi* plays a major role in the fluid movement of energy through the whole body. The energy channel connects the vitreous, kidneys, lungs, liver, and colon. If there is energy blockage, circulation suffers, and this leads to oxidative stress and inflammation. Stagnation can occur from stress or anxiety, and often leads to depression.[12] All of these conditions are risk factors for floaters. A liver detox may provide the key to their resolution.

EYE DROPS

One of my most recommended eye drops is the 15% MSM, or methylsulfonylmethane – a valuable agent for improving vitreous health. This is an organic, sulfur-containing nutrient that originates from microscopic plankton in the ocean. It is synthesized when a compound released by the plankton escapes into the atmosphere and reacts with the ozone and UV light.

MSM is then absorbed by plants and consumed by animals. Our bodies even contain MSM as a natural part of our blood plasma.

The health-promoting properties of MSM drops come from its sulfur. Many hormones, enzymes, antibodies, and antioxidants depend on it to properly carry out their functions. Sulfur also serves as a powerful anti-inflammatory, detoxification, and collagen-boosting agent.

Aside from a burning sensation that can last about ten seconds, MSM drops are completely safe, even in large doses, but I recommend starting with applications two to three times a day. You can use it to give yourself an eye massage or eye bath in the evenings along with a hexane-free castor oil in its pure form, making sure to keep the oil on the outside of the eyelids. These drops will prevent dry eye and dehydration, which can contribute to the development of new floaters.

BLUE LIGHT BLOCKERS

Blue light, especially from screens, increases eye strain and decreases circulation, often leading to floaters. Fortunately, you can protect your eyes in a number of ways, including blue light filtering glasses. In a 2020 study, participants reported that eye strain and dry eyes associated with screen exposure decreased when using blue light filters.[13]

EXERCISES FOR REDUCING FLOATERS

You'll find here a schedule for vision therapy exercises that most effectively tackles eye floaters. I encourage you to practice these exercises at least twice a day, once in the morning and once at night, and to challenge yourself to keep them up for 90 days. This long-term practice will help to relax your eyes, improve their circulation, and relieve stress. All of this will contribute to breaking up existing and preventing the accumulation of new floaters.

(Find the full description of these exercises on my website: https://www.drsamberne.com/eye-exercises/)

DAYS 1-7

- MSM Eye Massage
- N Breath and Palm Hum
- Sunning

DAYS 8-14

- Eye Dialogue
- Tongue Clock Palming

DAYS 15-21

- Long Swings
- N Breath and Palm Hum
- Eye Brain Body Fun

DAYS 22-30

- Figure 8 Eye Massage
- The Thumb Game

DAYS 31-37

- Sunning
- N Breath and Palm Hum
- Eye Dialogue

DAYS 38-46

- Yin Yang Charm
- Tongue Clock
- Figure 8 Eye Massage

DAYS 47-53

- Sunning
- MSM Eye Massage
- Eye Brain Body Fun

DAYS 54-60

- Long Swings
- The Thumb Game
- N Breath and Palm Hum

DAYS 61-69

- Eye Scan
- Sunning
- Figure 8 Eye Massage

DAYS 70-76

- Eye Dialogue
- Tongue Clock Palming
- MSM Eye Massage

DR. SAM BERNE

DAYS 77-81

- Long Swings
- The Thumb Game
- Yin Yang Charm

DAYS 82-90

- N Breath and Palm Hum
- Figure 8 Eye Massage
- Eye Brain Body Fun

FINAL THOUGHTS:

You may be overwhelmed after reading all the work it will take to reduce your floaters. Unfortunately, there is no magic bullet to eye health. It may take time, patience, and perseverance to figure out which methods will work best for you. But most of the changes are easily accessible and within your control, like diet and physical therapy exercises that you can do for a few minutes a day in the comfort of your own home.

If these recommendations have no effect on your floaters, I would suggest visiting a functional medicine specialist to explore some of the systemic, metabolic, and toxicity reasons in your body that might need healing. A doctor will also identify if there are issues with your eyes beyond your floaters.

Of course, going to the right doctor matters. Some doctors jump right to surgery to remove a problem before attempting alternatives that might heal the eye and prevent future ones. For example, a client of mine was referred to surgery after complaining to her doctor that she was seeing flashes. She came to see me before her scheduled surgery for a second opinion.

When I looked at her eyes, her retinas were still intact, but I could see a high presence of floaters and her vitreous was starting to come apart. Another big problem was that her contact lens prescription was about

40% stronger than it needed to be. After a week of using a reduced prescription for daily use, with another 15% reduction for work on the computer, she called to say her symptoms had improved.

We later went on to do vision therapy and I recommended some exercises to help her use both eyes together and develop more peripheral vision. I recommended she begin acupuncture and gave her some high potency antioxidant eye vitamins. We also explored color therapy. Within three months, the floaters and flashes of light had disappeared completely.

This is all to say, yet again, that you don't have to live out your diagnosis, and you have more options than just resorting to surgery. In concert with a trusted eye care professional who addresses the cause of your eye conditions, you can have more control over your eye health.

CHAPTER 2
CATARACTS

WHAT ARE CATARACTS?

Cataracts are the leading cause of preventable blindness. An estimated 65 million people globally suffer from cataracts,[1] at least 24 million in the United States alone, and experts estimate that number will surpass 50 million by 2050.[2] As you get older, if you find yourself diagnosed with cataracts, you're not alone – 90% of all people over the age of 65 will have cataracts.[3]

But remember: you don't have to live out your diagnosis, nor will you necessarily need surgery. Cataract formation is rooted in a metabolic problem in the eye, which means we can address and correct those problems through diet, eye exercises, and other lifestyle changes. You can take active steps towards preventing, reversing, and dissolving cataracts.

A cataract is an opaque spot that forms on the lens. The lens is positioned behind the colored iris and is the eye's main channel of directing light and forming clear retinal images. Cataracts on your lens create distortion and result in a cloudiness or haze in the vision.

As you get older, the lenses in your eyes become thicker, less transparent, and more rigid. When the proteins in the lens cells experience oxidative damage and poor circulation, they begin to clump together. Eventually, these clumps accumulate into a visible opaque spot – a cataract. The degree to which these spots can obscure your vision depends on the location and density of proteins. But if left untreated, they will continue to worsen.

WHAT ARE THE SYMPTOMS?

Symptoms of cataracts are blurry or hazy vision, a loss of color intensity, glare sensitivity, poor night vision, or a sudden worsening of your prescription. You may find yourself needing more light when reading. Maybe you struggle to make out street signs or notice your depth perception is off.

There are three types of cataracts, each with slightly different symptoms:

- Nuclear: This occurs in the center of the lens and affects your distance vision. This is the most common type of cataract. At first, with nuclear cataracts, your reading vision may seem to improve, but then get worse. With time, you might notice the cataract turning a denser yellow or even brown, making it harder to distinguish colors.
- Cortical: This takes shape around the periphery of the lens, in wedges or streaks like the spokes of a wheel. This is the second most common type of cataract. Cortical cataracts begin whitish around the edge of the lens, but as they progress, you'll notice the streaks moving closer towards the center, further obstructing your vision.[4]
- Posterior Subcapsular: This occurs at the back of the lens, right in the path of entering light. While this type of cataract is less common, it progresses much faster. The posterior subcapsular cataract will have the biggest impact on your reading and night vision. It typically causes halos around artificial light sources like headlights and streetlamps.

DISEASE PROGRESSION

If you think you might have cataracts, you should visit your doctor and begin discussing your options before they can develop any further. Given time, cataracts will only get worse, so the longer you avoid them, the more they will obscure your field of sight, and the more difficult they will be to correct.

Cataracts progress in three stages:

1. Early stage: This is where you may notice some subtle blurriness or light sensitivity. The cataracts may just be starting to form, but are not yet significantly affecting your visual acuity. If you suspect some of these early signs might indicate budding cataracts, a visit to your doctor now would be the best time to intervene with lifestyle changes to reduce them.
2. Moderate stage: Here is when you start to notice the reduction in your visual acuity. When vision problems begin to affect your daily life, this is a good sign you need to visit a doctor. When you go, be prepared to describe any instances of blurred vision, sensitivity to light, poor night vision, less color clarity, or even double vision.
3. Late stage: At this point, you need to have the cataract removed – lifestyle changes will not be enough to correct it. Late stage cataracts make it

difficult to do a significant amount of daily activities. If you avoid a doctor at this stage, you run the risk of permanent damage or blindness.

WHO IS AT RISK?

Most cataracts form as a result of oxidative stress, inflammation, and poor circulation in the eyes. As the aging process does lead to decreased oxygenation and hydration of the eye. This means that the older you are, the more susceptible you are to cataracts.

However, there are a number of factors that can increase your risk of developing them at a younger age.

Juvenile cataracts are those that develop within the first ten years of life, and pre-senile cataracts develop before 45 – but these are relatively uncommon. Some cataracts are genetic and may be present at birth, while others appear within the first year of life due to exposure to toxins. These are more likely in patients who have had eye injuries, radiation exposure, or other illnesses such as diabetes.[5]

People with diabetes are up to five times more likely to develop all types of cataracts, usually at an earlier age.[6] The eye's lens absorbs nutrients from the aqueous humor, a fluid containing oxygen and glucose found in the front of the eye. When this fluid has an excess of glucose, the lens swells. This causes poor circulation and cuts the tissue off from nutrients. In addition, the lens takes in glucose and converts it to sorbitol, but a build-up of sorbitol affects normal cell and protein activity in the lens, causing them to clump into cataracts.

Another major contributing factor is nutritional deficiency. Over 90% of Americans fall short of their daily requirements for many essential vitamins and minerals, including vitamins E, A, and C,[7] which are critical for eye health. This means there is a good chance your diet has a hand in forming your cataracts. The good news is that this is an almost entirely preventable risk factor: A 2000 study showed a 60% reduction in nuclear and cortical cataract risk for participants who reported taking a multivitamin supplement for over ten years.[8]

Poor gut health from a low fiber diet of highly processed foods might also be the culprit behind your cataracts. The microorganisms living in the intestine, which protect us from infection by bacterial pathogens, depend on fiber to do their job, and a lack of fiber in the diet is also linked to the development of chronic inflammatory diseases. One study showed that changing to a low fiber diet of highly processed foods reduced the number of gut bacteria, and caused persistent infection from low-grade inflammation and insulin resistance.[9] Chronic inflammation also cuts off circulation to the lens, which can lead to cataracts.

Excessive exposure to certain types of light can lead to a higher risk. Research suggests that UV light damages lens protein in the same way seen in cell damage from oxidative stress, promoting cataract development.[10] Chronic blue light exposure from digital devices and LED lights can also cause oxidative damage to the eye tissue,[11] leaving it susceptible to cataracts.

Other risk factors include obesity, hypertension, myopia (near-sightedness), trauma to the head or eyes, radiation exposure, drug and alcohol use, and certain inherited retinal degenerative diseases.

WHAT CAN I DO ABOUT THEM?

I recommend getting tested for cataracts at least once a year. Identifying the condition early is critical in treating and reversing it by non-surgical means.

A normal visit to the doctor for cataracts ends with, "Let's schedule you for surgery." You may ask for alternatives, but most doctors will brush off your concerns:

"Everybody gets cataracts. It's just what happens when you get old."

The standard approach to cataracts tells us to replace our damaged lens with a new one through surgery. And if cataracts have reached a certain point, that does become necessary. However, there are indeed many ways you can slow down or even reverse the condition long before that point.

Diet

Diet is at the top of my list as an underlying cause of most eye disorders, including cataracts.

As previously mentioned, cataracts form largely because of oxidative stress. That means that reactive oxygen particles called free radicals accumulate in the body faster than they can be cleared. A healthy eye cleans out this buildup when the mitochondria in the cells produce energy by absorbing and processing the nutrients we consume. The lens has no blood vessels running through it, so it relies on efficient nutrient absorption by the mitochondria to clear out the free radical damage. Inflammation similarly reduces the eye's ability to absorb nutrients. The good news is, both oxidative stress and inflammation can be reduced with positive dietary changes.

Incorporating more plants (fruits and vegetables) is key for supporting eye health and the reversal of cataracts. According to the CDC, only about 12% of adults in the U.S. meet their daily recommended intake of fruits, and only 9% get enough vegetables,[12] despite their many health benefits. Studies also show that fruits and vegetables reduce inflammation and may prevent chronic diseases[13] like diabetes that increase your risk of developing cataracts.

Think of the colors of the rainbow and try to vary the different colored vegetables you eat on a regular basis. The pigments in plants contain phytonutrients that give them their color, and each color contains different nutrients with varying health benefits. Chapter 9, Light, Color, and Vibrational Medicine for Healing the Eyes and Body, will address this topic in more depth, but there are some specific changes you can make to help with your cataracts.

Glutathione

Antioxidants reverse oxidative stress by removing free radicals from the body. The "master antioxidant" compound glutathione is my number one recommendation for addressing cataracts. Nearly every cell in the body contains glutathione. The body uses it in many processes, like tissue building and repair, synthesizing necessary chemicals and proteins, and immune function.

Studies have connected low glutathione levels to cataract development in mice.[14] A 2017 study on the effects on the skin of consuming oral glutathione showed significant anti-aging qualities including improved elasticity and the reduction of wrinkles.[15] As wrinkles and poor elasticity are signs of oxidative stress and inflammation, it follows that glutathione will similarly decrease the risks of cataracts. Studies have also shown glutathione to play a major part in the detoxification of heavy metal,[16] a build-up of which research shows increases several risk factors for developing cataracts.[17]

The recommended daily intake of glutathione is 15 mg, but I recommend a daily supplement of 240 mg per day, as research shows that supplementation can effectively raise body stores.[18]

Vitamins and Minerals
Sulfur: Sulfur-rich foods like garlic and onions can help boost the body's production of glutathione in the lens.

Sulfur sticks to the toxifying agents and heavy metals that the glutathione attracts and allows it to flush them out of the body. Sulfur also plays a role in improving the body's use of other vitamins and minerals.[19]

Vitamin C: Studies have suggested that vitamin C can assist in preventing cataracts[20] and in slowing their progression.[21] A 2016 study of people diagnosed with cataracts over 10 years showed a 33% reduced risk of progressive cataracts by adding vitamin C to the diet.[22]

Vitamin E: A powerful antioxidant with anti-inflammatory properties, vitamin E helps fight cataracts by reducing oxidative stress and improving circulation. Research has linked vitamin E to cataract prevention,[23] and a 2005 study suggested that long-term supplementation of vitamin E along with riboflavin (vitamin B2) and/or thiamine (vitamin B1) can decrease the progression of age-related lens opacification. In 2014, researchers concluded that a topical application of vitamin E as tocotrienol could delay the onset of cataracts and slow down their progression.[24]

Vitamin A: Another important antioxidant for eye health, more vitamin A can also form part of your prevention plan for future cataracts. According to the Blue Mountains Eye Study, vitamin A supplements, along with the

B vitamins, were associated with a reduced risk of nuclear or cortical cataracts.[25] A vitamin A intake, along with beta-carotene, is associated with a decreased risk for developing age-related cataracts.[26]

Carotenoids: Along with the benefits that come in combination with vitamin A, beta-carotene is a carotenoid that is an effective antioxidant for the lens. A randomized trial showed a 25% reduction in the risk of developing cataracts among smokers.[27] In addition, lutein and zeaxanthin are the only two carotenoids present in the actual lens of the eye.[28] Consumption of these nutrients may protect against cataract development.

Vitamin B2: The Blue Mountain Study also suggests that vitamin B2 (riboflavin) can protect against nuclear cataracts. Vitamin B2 takes part in many biochemical reactions, including oxidation-reduction with glutathione. Because of this, vitamin B2 deficiency plays an important role in cataract development.[29]

Vitamin D3: For overall eye health, it's a good idea to incorporate more vitamin D3 into your diet. Studies have suggested links between vitamin D and nuclear lens opacities.[30] One study in mice suggests that Vitamin D delays changes in metabolism and inflammation that reduce the risk of age-related eye diseases.[31] It may also function as an antioxidant.

Chromium: An essential trace element needed to maintain normal glucose metabolism, chromium blood levels in diabetics – among the most at risk for cataracts – are typically low. A 1992 study showed that chromium concentration in lenses with cataracts was about half or less that of clear lenses.[32]

Selenium: In studies, low selenium levels significantly predicted the formation of age-related cataracts.[33] Research suggests that it may prevent oxidative stress in the lens by strengthening its defensive system.[34]

Magnesium: Found in high concentrations in cell mitochondria, magnesium is the fourth most common mineral in the body. It plays an important part in maintaining lens homeostasis. Research suggests magnesium supplementation may prevent the onset and progression of cataracts.[35]

Zinc: The trace element zinc is present in high concentrations in eye tissue and plays an important role in maintaining normal eye function.[36] A recent study in rats showed the potential for zinc supplementation in slowing down the progression of cataracts in diabetics.[37]

Healthy Fats and Oils

Omega-3 oils reduce inflammation and keep eyes lubricated, nourished, and well-circulating,[38] creating an eye environment with reduced risk factors for cataracts. One study even found a significant inverse association with a high intake of omega-6 fatty acids and cataract development.[39]

Herbs and Spices

Eye-healthy herbs and spices include cilantro, ginger, turmeric, and peppermint.

Gut Health

A healthy bacterial environment within the human gastrointestinal tract is necessary for proper digestion, nutrient production, detoxification, pathogen protection, and immune system regulation.[40] Gut health can be harmed by pesticides, heavy metal toxicity, mold, and candida.

But the largest part of promoting healthy gut bacteria involves diet. It's particularly important to avoid foods that lead to inflammation, including *animal products, processed foods, alcohol, sugar, soy, and gluten.* In a UK study, vegetarians had a 30% lower risk of developing cataracts than those who ate high quantities of animal products, while vegans had a 40% lower risk![41]

Probiotics or pre-probiotic fiber supplements can improve gut health, but I recommend discussing this with your functional medicine doctor and making dietary changes first.

Eye Drops

Several types of eye drops can slow or reverse the development of cataracts. Oclumed is an all-natural cataract-reversing eye drop that contains both glutathione and vitamin C and helps improve eye circulation. It can be used for three months, four to six times a day. There is some indication that NAC carnosine eye drops may prevent or reduce the progression of cataracts, but more research is needed into this effect.[42] Optique and Simalison are homeopathic eye drops I recommend.

I also recommend the use of 15% methylsulfonylmethane (MSM) eye drops. While MSM drops will not reverse your cataracts, the hydrating effect will allow for more cell permeability. This makes both nutritional changes and other eyedrops more effective. Use the MSM eye drop before using other drops because they will make your cells more permeable and receptive. In combination, they can work to remove opacities and dissolve your cataracts.

Lifestyle Changes

There are some general changes we can apply to our lifestyle that can support cataract prevention. Exercise reduces the risk and potentially reverses type 2 diabetes,[43] a risk factor for cataracts. Quit smoking, taking drugs, or drinking alcohol to reduce oxidative stress. Practice mindfulness exercises to reduce overall body stress, and take any measures you can to reduce the visual stress caused by blue and UV light. Hundreds of my patients have reduced their cataracts just by changing their diet, doing some detoxification processes, and reducing their stress levels.

IF YOU NEED SURGERY

Once cataracts start to interfere with your daily activities, it becomes much more difficult, even impossible, to dissolve them through diet and lifestyle changes. At this point, it's time for surgery.

The surgery itself is an outpatient procedure that typically takes less than an hour. The doctor applies a local anesthetic to numb the area around your eye, and you may get a sedative to relax, but you're awake through the brief process. The surgeon will remove the cloudy lens and replace it with an artificial one known as an intraocular lens (IOL), a new piece of hardware that becomes a permanent part of your eye.

You'll need to choose an intraocular lens before your procedure. Here are some of the different types of lenses:

- Standard: Otherwise known as the "monofocal" lens, this choice is good for long-distance vision needs like watching TV or driving. When patients have other eye conditions, like glaucoma, diabetic retinopathy, or macular degeneration, this is the most common lens choice.
- Bifocal: Also called the "dual focus" lens, this choice corrects both distance and near vision. However, common side effects can include double vision or halos of light while driving at night.
- Toric: This choice corrects distance only and is a special lens for astigmatism.
- Accommodating lens: The "crystalens," as it is called, allows patients to shift their focus various distances through this lens's flexible hinges.

Some patients may still end up needing reading glasses for small print, and this choice is not for astigmatism.
- Aspheric: This lens can help improve contrast in situations of intense light or darkness.
- Monovision: This implant technique uses a standard lens with a different focusing power in each eye so the patient has no need for glasses after surgery. For example, the dominant eye would be corrected for distance vision while the non-dominant was corrected for near. I don't recommend this lens because it reduces depth perception and makes it difficult for both eyes to work together.
- EDOF: This IOL has an invisible bifocal built into it, though this can make it difficult for the patient to aim their eyes when focusing.

Your IOL is a forever decision, so carefully consider your options. More complicated IOL designs can create more confusion for the brain, but the surgeon likely will only consider the optical mechanisms, not how they interact with the brain.

When you get the operation, make sure to tell the doctor to correct both eyes for distance instead of different corrections in each eye. One client I knew got monovision in her IOLs for cataract surgery and she was a mess – mental confusion, difficulty reading. I got her contact lenses to help correct the eyes for distance so they could start working together and she immediately felt the relaxation in her nervous and neuromuscular system.

I recommend you ask for a single vision lens correcting both eyes for distance to support eye-brain communication and depth perception. If you're thinking about bifocal or astigmatism lenses, think again: It will be much harder for your eyes and brain to figure out how to use them.

If you use digital devices often, you may require a higher quality lens with blue-light blocking filtration, but your budget might set limits on what you can afford. If you opt for a less expensive model without a blue-light filter, this can result in macular degeneration, so at least invest in a pair of blue-blocking glasses if not the more expensive lens filter to avoid exchanging one eye condition for another.

PREPARING FOR SURGERY

Even once you've decided on surgery, chosen an IOL, and scheduled date, you can still take actions to improve the results. Dietary and lifestyle changes during the period leading up to your surgery will help speed up the healing process and reintegration of eye function with its new hardware after your surgery. Here are some ways you can be better prepared:

Traditional Chinese Medicine (TCM)

Seeing a TCM practitioner before your cataract surgery can help improve circulation in your meridians, and thus in your eyes. Meridians are the pathways in our bodies that allow our life force as well as other bodily fluids to flow smoothly, indicating wellness. Blockages, on the other hand, result in pain and illness. Starting at the big toe, the liver meridian travels up the leg and to the chest, where it connects with the liver and gallbladder before continuing up to the eyes. This meridian is the main pathway for eye health.

Acupuncture points on the skin allow the practitioner to access the meridians and clear any blockages. According to TCM expert Dr. Andy Rosenfarb, "Acupuncture is clearly an effective means of managing most chronic and degenerative eye diseases [with] measurable improvement in approximately 70-80% of all cases treated."[44] Start acupuncture treatment a month before your surgery and go weekly to get your meridians working again.

Psychological Preparation

Many patients experience psychological stress regarding either the formation of cataracts or the surgery to remove them. If you have a lot of emotional baggage around the surgery, you'll still be carrying it around after. Clear up your feelings before you go under and those feelings will be less likely to linger. When we believe therapy can work, it does, so go into therapy believing it will support your cataract surgery recovery and it will.

Find a therapist – craniosacral or one who focuses on clearing emotional blocks – and clear up the psycho-emotional energies around your cataracts. I perform craniosacral therapy with my patients and have seen it release this negative energy. It's a game-changer in how well the patient does with the surgery.

Boost Your Immune System

Start taking probiotics or pre-probiotic fiber to get your gut healthy. Keep it healthy with a high fiber diet of plant-based foods full of colorful fruits and veggies high in antioxidants. Surgery will slow down your dietary absorption, but a diet high in antioxidants will improve cellular absorption, metabolism, and waste removal in the eyes.

. . .

Avoid foods that cause inflammation and work with a naturopathic doctor to reduce stress and balance your systemic and metabolic levels. Up your vitamin C intake along with the master antioxidant glutathione for lens health, as well as other nutrients for eye health. Use homeopathic eye drops a couple of weeks before surgery. If you follow these tips, you'll find better resiliency in health to come through your cataract surgery successfully.

WHAT HAPPENS AFTER SURGERY?

The swelling will go down after about 48 hours and you should quickly feel better, but even after recovering from surgery, there are steps that you can take to ensure your eyes stay healthy.

What To Avoid - First 48 hours after surgery:

- driving
- exposure to bright lights or electronic devices
- rubbing your eyes
- hanging or bending upside down

What To Avoid - First week after surgery:

- strenuous lifting or exercise
- swimming in pools or soaking in hot tubs

Blue Light Blockers

Your natural lens, which was removed during surgery, had a blue-blocking agent that protected your macula. This leaves you vulnerable to macular degeneration. In most cases, unless you've ordered a special IOL, the lens they put into your eyes for cataract surgery doesn't. Your eye is much more susceptible to blue light damage without its natural protection. To protect your macula, I recommend two things: supplementing with lutein and wearing blue-filtering glasses for all digital devices, including TV.

Eye Drops

It's common for doctors to recommend eye drops post-surgery to reduce inflammation, dryness, and redness, and prevent infection, but most of those they prescribe contain preservatives or vasoconstrictors that can worsen macular degeneration. Instead, once you have a clean bill of health, start using natural or homeopathic eye drops. I recommend a hexane-free, organic castor oil eye drop or MSM to be protective and reduce inflammation.

Essential Oils

Several essential oils can boost recovery from cataract surgery.

- Sweet fennel, carrot seed, and frankincense: Keep these oils away from your eyes, but put a drop above your hairline, by the ears, your mouth or anywhere else a safe distance from the general anatomy of the eyes. Apply them one at a time in layers, one over the other. This will surround the eyes with a boost of oxygenation and hydration and can eliminate some of the effects of the anesthesia from surgery.
- Neroli oil: This essential oil from the orange blossom plant has antibacterial properties and a highly oxygenating and hydrating effect. One study in pregnant women demonstrated its calming effects,[45] and a 2015 animal study showed its potential for treating pain and inflammation.[46] Put four to six drops onto a cool, wet washcloth, and place it over your eyes for five to ten minutes, every day for five days.
- Lavender oil: Well-known for its calming, soothing, and balancing effects, lavender oil also reduces anxiety and promotes a restful night's

sleep, even after surgery.[47] Lavender is also an effective stress reducer.[48] A 2012 study of lavender oil treatment post-surgery suggests it can even reduce the need for opioids in managing pain.[49] Put three drops onto a cotton ball and place it in your pillowcase before bed to benefit from the nighttime inhalation of this soothing oil.

Diet

Of course, I recommend sticking to an anti-inflammatory diet of whole, unprocessed foods, colorful fruits and veggies, and eye-healthy nutrients. Boosting our eye nutrition is about reducing metabolic stress, and anything you can do to reduce visual stress is helpful for healing your eyes after surgery.

Post-Surgery Eye Exercises

I recommend at least two weeks of low-stress eye exercises. Even though your cataract is gone, it developed in the first place for a reason. Building resilience in your eyes after surgery will help to prevent eye conditions from developing in the future so you can keep your sight until 100!

- Palming: Invented by New York ophthalmologist Dr. William Bates, the practice of palming relaxes and refreshes your eyes, reducing their dependency on glasses. Palming can be done lying down or sitting up, but make sure your back and neck are straight, and shoulders relaxed. Rub your hands quickly together for about 10 seconds so the heat can draw out the tension from your eyes. Softly cup your warm hands over your closed eyes without making contact with the eyelids. You can rest your elbows on the table in front of you. Breath slowly and relax the body and the eyes. Do this anywhere from two to five minutes, six times a day, or whenever you need to relax. When you've finished, slowly take your hands away. You'll feel refreshed, and the world will appear much clearer and brighter!
- Thumb rotations – This exercise is a great practice for any eye disease. By moving your eyes in a relaxed, effortless manner, you develop greater eye-mind-body awareness and improve ocular function. Start by standing up and cover one eye with your hand. Hold the other outstretched in front of you with your thumb facing up and trace a circular motion in both directions. Follow the thumb with your open eye. Remember to breathe, blink, and feel the eye muscles stretching. Do this practice for two minutes a day on both eyes, every day.

EYE EXERCISES FOR CATARACT REVERSAL

Below is my cataract-specific eye exercise protocol for those of you who haven't yet undergone surgery. Use these if you see the signs of cataracts beginning to form and want to reverse and heal them. These eye exercises are designed to improve hydration, circulation, and flexibility of the eye to combat the build-up of oxidative stress causing cataracts in the first place. I encourage you to practice these exercises at least twice a day, once in the morning and once at night, and to challenge yourself to keep them up for 90 days. All of this will contribute to reversing and preventing cataracts.

(Find the full description of these exercises on my website: https://www.drsamberne.com/eye-exercises/)

DAYS 1-7

- MSM Eye Massage
- N Breath and Palm Hum
- Long Swings

DAYS 8-14

- Long Swings

- Eye Scan
- Tongue Clock Palming

DAYS 15-21

- Yin Yang Chart
- Eye Dialogue

DAYS 22-30

- MSM Eye Massage
- Eye Scan

DAYS 31-37

- Eye Scan
- N Breath and Palm Hum

DAYS 38-46

- Long Swings
- Tongue Clock Palming

DAYS 47-53

- MSM Eye Massage
- Eye Dialogue
- Yin Yang Chart

DAYS 54-60

- Long Swings
- Eye Scan
- N Breath and Palm Hum

DAYS 61-69

- MSM Eye Massage
- Eye Scan

DAYS 70-76

- Eye Dialogue
- Tongue Clock Palming

DR. SAM BERNE

DAYS 77-81

- Long Swings
- Eye Scan
- Yin Yang Chart

DAYS 82-90

- N Breath and Palm Hum
- MSM Eye Massage

Visit my website, https://www.drsamberne.com, to take advantage of the wealth of up-to-date information, including hundreds of video blogs on different conditions and 90-day EyeClarity protocols for reversing them. You can also find all eye exercise protocols described in this book at: https://www.drsamberne.com/eye-exercises/.

CHAPTER 3
MACULAR DEGENERATION

WHAT IS MACULAR DEGENERATION?

Age-related Macular Degeneration (AMD) is the leading cause of blindness in people over 60. It affects over 11 million Americans, and experts estimate that number will double by 2050. One-third of people will develop MD in their lifetime, and the estimated global cost of visual impairment due to AMD is $343 billion, including $255 in direct health care costs.[1]

Yet despite these serious costs to our wallets and health, when your doctor recognizes the signs of AMD, they say "Let's watch it and see what happens." As early as optometry school they learn to tell their patients that AMD is simply an aging problem. They prescribe a regimen of medications called "Anti-VEGF," which may slow down the symptoms, but improves vision for only one in three people, can cause anxiety and discomfort, and never cures the condition. They tell you, "There's not much else we can do."

But a diagnosis of "wait and see" until it gets bad enough to take action is not something you have to accept. The progression of AMD is avoidable through natural remedies that reduce root causes, not cover them up by only addressing the symptoms. If you focus on restoring the imbalance in your eyes that caused the macular degeneration, you can heal your macula and restore your vision.

Macular degeneration occurs in the macula at the center of the retina, the thin layer of tissue at the back of the eye. It takes up less than 1% of the retina, but it is critical to our ability to see most color and to see enough detail to read and recognize faces. While the other 99% of our retina processes vision in our periphery, the macula contains photoreceptors that help us focus our straight-ahead vision into sharp, clear, colorful images.

If we zoom into the eye anatomy even closer, we would see the macula in different layers. The tiny blood vessels, or microcapillaries, feed it nutrients from the very back of the ocular cavity (eye socket). Next, a thin layer of vascular tissue called the Bruch's membrane separates those blood vessels from the retinal pigment epithelium (RPE). The RPE is a single layer of highly pigmented cells that form the final blood-retina barrier. Preventing the progression of AMD involves the health of all three of these layers.

The macula has the highest metabolic needs of all retinal tissue and relies on the indirect supply of nutrients from the surrounding blood vessels for nourishment. That reliance on microcapillaries means that it is very susceptible to oxidative damage. Oxidative damage occurs when oxygen particles called free radicals accumulate in the body faster than they can be cleared. A healthy eye cleans out this buildup when the mitochondria in the cells produce energy by absorbing and processing the nutrients we consume. But a build-up of waste in the retinal microcapillaries dries out and weakens the macular tissue, while cutting it off from the nutrients it needs to eliminate that excess build-up.

TYPES OF MACULAR DEGENERATION

There are two types of AMD, dry and wet. There are slight differences in what you might notice that would distinguish which of the two types of AMD is affecting your vision, but visiting your doctor is the only way to confirm your condition.

. . .

Dry AMD represents up to 90% of the diagnosed cases of AMD. Yellow deposits of lipids and protein waste called *drusen* form in the Bruch's membrane naturally with age, but when they grow too large or in great quantities, they can damage and kill the macular tissue. As cellular function in the macula declines, vision becomes more blurred. In rare cases, dry AMD can result in serious vision damage.

In one out of 10 cases, dry AMD will progress to *wet AMD* and cause even more vision loss. When oxygenation and waste build up in the macula, abnormal blood vessels can begin to develop to attempt to compensate. But without sufficient nutrients and circulation, these abnormal blood vessels grow weak and are prone to damage. They can begin to bleed and leak fluid through the Bruch's membrane and into the RPE (which is why the condition is called "wet"). This causes the macula to bulge and create visual distortions.

Even in the early stages, dry AMD can change to wet very suddenly. In very rare cases, wet AMD can even occur before or instead of the dry condition. Wet AMD accounts for 90% of legal blindness. While less common, it is a much more aggressive condition and can progress rapidly.

SYMPTOMS AND PROGRESSION

Symptoms of AMD include visual distortion, inflammation, and a loss of visual detail. First, you may notice lines looking wavy or blurry objects that never clear up. There can be a splotch or blotchiness in the center of your vision. You may feel like it's coming on quite suddenly, but the condition has probably already been going on for a while.

Generally, AMD progresses along four stages:

1. Early stage:

At this point, you may not have any symptoms or vision loss, but the damage has already begun. An eye doctor would be able to examine and detect the size and number of drusen in an eye exam, but at this point, they will only document them and monitor their growth.

2. Intermediate stage:

By now, you have many medium-sized drusen and potentially one or more large drusen accumulating in your macula. Merging or large drusen can indicate a higher risk of disease progression. You may need more light to complete daily activities that require focus or notice a blurred spot in the middle of your vision. In the intermediate stage, vision loss is still possible, but you can generally still live your life very effectively.

3. Advanced stage:

In advanced AMD, light-sensitive cells in the macular tissue begin to break down. Weak, abnormal blood vessels can start to grow underneath the retina. By this stage, symptoms can severely impact your daily life, including:

- blurred vision or straight lines that look distorted or wavy
- light sensitivity
- difficulty reading or writing
- blind spots at the center of your vision
- difficulty distinguishing colors
- reduced depth perception

4. End stage:

This final stage of AMD is permanent vision loss that can no longer be treated by eye injections or surgery. People who advance into this stage of AMD would be considered "legally blind" and eligible for the corresponding government benefits.

WHO IS AT RISK?

As the name "Age-related Macular Degeneration" suggests, age is the primary risk factor in developing the disease. There are two underlying reasons that age leads to AMD. First, as you get older, your body becomes less able to combat the free radicals that cause oxidative stress, which breaks down macular photoreceptors. This leads to poor eye circulation and the buildup of drusen or abnormal blood vessel growth. Second, more and larger drusen deposits naturally accumulate over time.

How drusen deposits form is still unclear, but research suggests that RPE cells discard unwanted proteins and lipids into the Bruch's membrane. Minerals like calcium, phosphate, zinc, and iron, then stick to that RPE waste, forming clumps of drusen.[2] Drusen formation is a natural process, but in higher quantities or larger sizes, drusen deposits may indicate the early stage of AMD. Healthy eyes with good circulation, hydration, and oxygenation have the mechanisms to clear this waste accumulation. But age, along with other risk factors, diminishes this capacity.

Obviously, we can't stop the aging process, but certain factors cause the aging process to lead to poorer health. If we address the risk factors described below, we reduce the likelihood that aging will lead to poor eye health.

Oxidative Stress

Oxidative stress is a major contributor to AMD. When free radicals accumulate in the eyes, they cannot function properly. In both wet and dry AMD, the macula is cut off from essential nutrients. This further inhibits the eye's ability to eliminate metabolic waste build-up, causing more oxidative damage and further compounding the condition.

Of course, the body's capacity to do this with age declines, but other factors, such as exposure to environmental pollutants, heavy metal toxicities, reactions to certain drugs or chemical solutions, cigarette smoke, alcohol use, and even some cooking processes can result in the excess production of free radicals.[3]

UV and Blue Light

In dry AMD, light is one of the main oxidative factors in degrading the macula's photoreceptor cells. The visible light spectrum, particularly blue light, can cause significant oxidative stress in the RPE.[4] UV radiation has identified as a risk factor for human retinal health, especially for people over 40.[5]

Cataract surgery can put your eyes at further risk for this damage. The eye's natural lens has some protection against blue light, but the artificial intraocular lens (IOL) implanted in surgery may not. If you are scheduled for cataract surgery, you still have time to ask your surgeon to put a blue-light filter in your IOL. If you've already had surgery, and you're still using the computer or watching TV as you did before, you need to add a layer of blue-light protection to keep your macula from degenerating.

Smoking

Cigarette smoke contains high concentrations of oxidizing chemicals and metals involved in the oxidation and damage of cellular proteins. It compounds free radical overproduction and cell death in the body.[6] With the smoke so close to your face, this oxidative stress invariably affects the eyes, so it's no surprise that studies have linked smoking with a higher risk of AMD.[7]

Multifocal Progressive Lenses

Otherwise known as the "no-line bifocal" or progressive lenses, those glasses you use to improve your vision may actually be hurting it in the long run. When you use multifocal lenses, they reduce your vision to a tiny sliver in the center of the lens – your macula. Instead of the work of focusing the eyes being distributed across the entire lens of the eye, the macula bears the entire strain. This increased stress can eventually wear out the macula. High intensity focusing, such as looking at a computer or phone screen, is particularly wearing.

Chronic Diseases

If you already have a chronic issue, like cardiovascular disease, hypertension, chronic fatigue syndrome, or diabetes, check with your eye doctor to make sure your macula is healthy. Any condition that compromises the immune system reduces circulation and nutrition. Wet AMD can often be a pre-diabetic condition, and could actually be causing the development of abnormal blood in the macula, so if you're diagnosed with one of these conditions, check for the other.

Over the Counter or Prescription Drugs

Several types of drugs increase sensitivity to light, which may cause chemical modification of the eye tissue and lead to retinal and macular hemorrhages. These include:

- Non-steroidal anti-inflammatory drugs (NSAIDs), such as ibuprofen, aspirin, ketoprofen, flurbiprofen, and naproxen sodium[8]
- Tranquilizers[9]
- Sulfa drugs[10]
- Antidepressants[11]

- Antihistamines[12]
- Clonidine (used to treat high blood pressure)[13]
- Plaquenil (used to treat arthritis)[14]
- Birth control pills[15]

High Cholesterol

While we may think of it as the "good" cholesterol, studies are showing that we may need to be concerned about high levels of high-density lipoproteins (HDL). A 2004 study found a link between high HDL cholesterol levels and a higher risk of AMD.[16] A 2019 study found an association with elevated HDL levels and increased drusen accumulation, enhancing your risk of developing dry AMD.[17]

WHEN TO VISIT A DOCTOR

Since AMD may progress slowly and without symptoms, it's important to visit your ophthalmologist regularly as you age. The earlier you can detect AMD, the more effective lifestyle changes can be at reversing and curing it.

If you do notice any symptoms of AMD, especially abnormalities at the center of your vision, you should visit your doctor immediately. Make sure you tell your doctor about any pharmaceutical drugs that you're taking to see if their side effects might be underlying your AMD.

It's possible that your vision distortion might also be from macular pucker, which is a different condition involving scar tissue in the macula, but it has many of the same symptoms as AMD. The underlying causes of pucker and AMD are different, though, so the process for fixing each condition would be, too. Visiting a doctor to confirm your eye health first is the best way to move on to treating it.

Your doctor will perform several different tests to determine if you have AMD.

1. The Amsler Grid Test:

Even before going to the doctor, you can do the Amsler Grid test on yourself at home. It's basically a series of lines made into a square grid with a dark dot at the center that you can download and print for free on the internet. Cover one eye and hold the grid about 14 inches from your face while focusing on the central dot. If you notice any curvature or horizontal, vertical, or diagonal waviness around the straight lines, this may be a sign of macular degeneration.

2. Fluorescein Angiography:

Next, the doctor will look for abnormal blood vessel growth in the retina or macula to determine the risk for wet AMD. They inject a yellow dye into your body, which travels through the blood vessels and into the eye, where a camera captures retinal images as the dye passes through its microcapillaries.

3. Optical Coherence Tomography:

In this next test, a machine will scan your eye for detailed images of the retina and macula, which your doctor can evaluate to identify any abnormalities.

WHAT CAN I DO ABOUT IT?

Once your doctor has determined that you have AMD, it's time to decide on your course of treatment.

The most common treatment for dry AMD is the AREDS2 supplement formula a combination of vitamin C, vitamin E, beta-carotene, copper, lutein, zeaxanthin, and zinc. This was developed by following the 2013 Age-Related Eye Disease Study 2 and has been proven effective in slowing the progression of AMD. [18]

But otherwise, unless it worsens into wet AMD, doctors often say there is little else they can do.

Surgery for dry AMD is a very rare procedure only used in cases of geographic atrophy – an advanced condition where retinal cells die. The doctor removes the eye's natural lens and replaces it with a miniature telescope behind the iris, which enlarges and focuses images on healthier areas in the retina. Of course, an implanted telescope in your eye will come with side effects, including reduced peripheral vision, corneal swelling, double vision, or infection.[19]

Previously, some doctors would recommend hot laser surgery to burn and seal the bleeding vessels in the back of the eye from wet AMD. But the laser burn itself left a space where the patient could no longer see. Further, the bleed can come back, or a new lesion can develop around the site of the laser treatment.[20] There is also a cold laser procedure, with its own risks, such as cell loss in the treated area.

Now, a typical treatment for wet AMD is through eye injections of anti-vascular endothelial growth factor drugs (anti-VEGF). Vascular endothelial growth factor (VEGF) is a signal protein produced in cells that plays a major role in controlling the development and progression of choroidal neovascularization (CNV), or abnormal blood vessel growth in the choroid of the eye. Studies have shown that taking anti-VEGF can help maintain visual acuity in patients with wet AMD.[21] At the same time, regular anti-VEGF injections throughout a patient's lifetime can encourage retinal and choroidal atrophy, eventually reducing visual acuity anyway. It can also impose inhibitive financial and medical burdens, and researchers have been searching for more efficient treatments, like gene therapy, as alternatives.[22]

Of course, my recommendation is to avoid surgery and pharmaceutical drugs that treat the problem, but leave behind the cause – and create some additional side effects in the process. As we've seen, the underlying cause of macular degeneration is a lack of oxygen, hydration, and antioxidants reaching the eye and leading to drusen formation, so addressing those root causes is key.

Natural ways to manage and reduce the drusen of dry AMD and the CNV that cause wet AMD still exist at any stage of the condition, but they take dedication and attention to all areas of our systemic health, including diet, exercise, and other lifestyle changes. The sooner you start to put in the work with these methods, the sooner you can heal your macular degeneration.

DIET

Diet is one of the main branches of holistic lifestyle changes that I recommend to address AMD. Again, think of the colors of the rainbow and try to vary the different colored fruits and vegetables you eat on a regular basis. The pigments in plants contain phytonutrients that give them their color, and each color contains different nutrients with varying health benefits. Chapter 8, Nutrition Tips for Healthy Eyes, will address this topic in more depth, but there are some specific changes you can make to help with your AMD.

One of the key ingredients that make these rainbow-colored plant foods so effective is their high levels of antioxidants. With oxidation being such a dominant force in causing AMD, the more antioxidants we can consume in our diet, the better.

Carotenoids, found in many red and orange foods, are effective antioxidants for the lens, particularly if you have a build-up of toxicities due to chronic inflammation or excessive UV or blue light exposure. An antioxidant blend plus zinc, copper, and omega-3 fatty acids has been linked to a 25% reduced risk for the development and progression of AMD.[23]

• • •

Other fruits and vegetables can also help to detoxify the body. Not only are apples a good source of vitamins C and fiber, in one study, apple peels showed the potential to actually purify water.[24] Celery is also a good source of fiber and vitamin C, as well as powerful antioxidants to combat free radicals. In animal studies, celery seed extract showed the potential to treat diabetes and improve the capabilities of antioxidant enzymes.[25] A 2015 animal study demonstrated the effects of celery seed oil extract on restoring liver function and detoxifying the body.[26]

Maybe an entirely plant-based diet isn't for you, but studies show that a compromise is also effective in improving eye health. The Mediterranean diet is best known for being heart-healthy, but new research suggests it also reduces the risk of AMD by 41%.[27] This diet is high in plant-based foods fish and low in meat and dairy, with olive oil as the primary source of fat.

Eat more nori seaweed, cod, and pasture-fed eggs for dietary iodine. A 2014 study found participants with higher levels of urinary iodine showed healthier maculas, less edema, and less swelling.[28]

Make sure to focus on healthy fats from sources like avocado, walnuts, pecans, and hazelnuts. Get plenty of soluble fiber from beans, lentils, or peas. Balance out your cholesterol levels, avoid trans-fatty acids, and don't overdo it on HDL fats.

Foods to Avoid

While incorporating healthy foods into your diet, be sure to avoid or minimize foods that cause inflammation, as researchers have identified strong links between systemic inflammation and AMD.[29]

High consumption of omega-6 fatty acids can lead to chronic diseases associated with inflammation.[30] This means you should avoid foods like potato chips and crackers that are fried in canola, soybean, or sunflower oil.

Sugar can also cause digestive problems and inflammation that inevitably have an effect on the eyes. Not only will ditching sugar reduce your risk of obesity and chronic diseases like diabetes – which increase your risk of developing AMD – cutting sugar from your diet enhances your fitness level, improves sleep, and decreases the effects of anxiety and depression. The only thing you have to lose in cutting sugar from your diet is an addiction.

• • •

Foods For Gut Health

Poor gut health from a low fiber diet of highly processed foods might also be the culprit behind your AMD. The microorganisms living in the intestine, which protect us from infection by bacterial pathogens, depend on fiber to do their job. A lack of fiber in the diet is also linked to the development of chronic inflammatory diseases. One study showed that changing to a low fiber diet of highly processed foods reduced the number of gut bacteria, and caused persistent infection from low-grade inflammation and insulin resistance. Chronic inflammation also cuts off circulation to the eye, which can lead to AMD.

Studies have shown the role of gut microbiota in intraocular inflammation and have even identified a personalized microbiome in the aqueous humor of human and animal eyes. Researchers have connected an increased bacterial content with drusen deposits in cases of AMD.[31] In a 2020 animal study, researchers found improving the gut microbiome resulted in reduced inflammation and improved retinal health.[32]

Take probiotics or gut cleansing enzymes to clean up and improve your dietary absorption and reduce the body's inflammatory response. A smoothie or juice cleanse can create a lot of great enzymatic gut action.

• • •

Supplements

Making sure that you get all the nutrients vital to eye health in your diet can be overwhelming or even impossible for some. Fortunately, there are many that you can take as supplements that are just as effective. The AREDS2 formulation, mentioned earlier, is the gold standard for slowing the progression of AMD, but individual nutrients can also be supplemented.

Carotenoids

Lutein and zeaxanthin are two carotenoids that exist in higher concentrations in eye tissue, particularly the macula, than anywhere else in the body. The yellow pigment, zeaxanthin, surrounds the macula. Lutein plays a functional role in eye tissue homeostasis.[33] Both carotenoid antioxidants protect the macula from UV and blue light, which degrade the macular cells. Take 16 mg of lutein and four to six mg of zeaxanthin daily to improve eye health and reverse the damage of MD.

Another carotenoid antioxidant making waves is astaxanthin. Astaxanthin is a marine carotenoid that our bodies can't produce, but we can consume in dietary sources like pink seafood or microalgae. Animal and human studies have been demonstrating increasing evidence of astaxanthin's benefits, including protection against cardiovascular disease, reducing oxidative stress and inflammation, and its antioxidant capacity has been shown to be even more potent than vitamin E and beta-carotene in trapping free radicals.[34] Astaxanthin also demonstrates powerful effects on eye health. A 2012 study in mice found that astaxanthin reduces retinal cell death in cases of diabetic retinopathy and improves oxidative stress markers.[35] We're also learning that this antioxidant shields the eye against the oxidative damage of blue and UV light and helps eliminate free radicals. In a 2020 study, astaxanthin inhibited cell death caused by blue light exposure, suppressed the production of oxidative stress biomarkers, and reduced mitochondrial damage in retinal cells.[36]

Seniors who use their digital devices throughout the day should consider supplementing with astaxanthin. I recommend 12 to 15 mg per day. You can find natural supplements, but make sure they contain phospholipids, which help with the absorption of antioxidants throughout the body and into the eyes.[37]

Omega-3 Fatty Acids

A 2007 animal study found omega-3s to protect against the development and progression of retinal deterioration, or retinopathy.[38] Supplement omega-3s with fish or algae oil, and make sure to eat healthy fats from sources like avocados, coconut oil, nuts, seeds, and MCT oils.

Vitamin D

Vitamin D plays a major role in bone mineral homeostasis, and studies have shown a connection between vitamin D levels and the incidence of chronic diseases. Vitamin D protects against oxidative stress in retinal cells, reduces a major component of drusen, and inhibits inflammation – all of which show its potential in preventing or treating early AMD.[39]

Vitamin B12

Vitamin B12 is vital to the central nervous system, blood cells, and DNA synthesis. You can get more B12 from animal food sources or fortified foods like cereals and nutritional yeast. One study in women showed a 30-40% reduced risk of developing AMD when supplementing with a combination of folic acid and vitamins B6 and B12. It's recommended to take 1000 micrograms of B12 per day.[40]

LIFESTYLE CHANGES

In addition to reducing systemic inflammation caused by dietary factors, you can take additional steps to reduce the lifestyle and environmental factors causing stress and exacerbating the problem.

Exercise

Exercise is beneficial to your eyes as well as your overall health! Cardiovascular fitness is important in reducing AMD. Thirty minutes of aerobic exercise a day improves circulation throughout the body – including the eyes! Eye physical therapy exercises like the ones described below help open the vision and create new pathways to seeing. They maximize the eye's ability to modify, change, and adapt both structure and function throughout life and in response to experience.

UV and Blue Light Protection

UV and blue light are major causes of oxidative stress and eye strain, so wear blue-blocking lenses on digital devices and UV-blocking sunglasses outside between the hours of 9:00 AM and 5:00 PM.

Quit Smoking

Quitting smoking may significantly slow the rate of your macular degeneration.

Alternative Therapies

Chinese medicine and acupuncture can be beneficial for general systemic health and overall eye health. A practitioner can open up the meridians that go to the eyes and get more energy to your macula. The liver is the primary organ that innervates the eye, so you can also try methods to increase the available energy in your liver, like a detoxification program.

Get some regular bodywork to improve your lymphatic and circulatory systems. Craniosacral therapy can improve the cerebral spinal fluid, blood, and lymph flow, not just in the eyes, but throughout the whole body.

Other Methods

Using one distance lens for everything is going to narrow your vision and put all the stress on your maculas, but the bigger the window you look through, the more you're accessing other parts of the retina. Reduce your progressive lenses and get separate single vision lenses for computer work and reading to keep your maculas from wearing out.

Chapter 8, Light, Color, and Movement To Improve Eye Health and Vision, will address how color therapy, or "chromotherapy," can help improve macular health. This practice is helpful for the photoreceptors of the eyes, as well as mitigating stress, which can weaken your eye systems.

• • •

If you use an eye drop to hydrate and oxygenate your eyes, avoid using ones like Visine that have preservatives or vasoconstrictors, which can end up making macular degeneration worse. Instead, I recommend homeopathic drops (Simalysan or Optique) and 5% MSM eye drops.

EYE EXERCISES FOR MACULAR DEGENERATION

To heal any macular problem, it's necessary to open up our vision – to use other parts of the retina and take the stress off the macula. The macula makes up less than 1% of the retina, but it's our central focal point for bringing light into our vision. However, retraining the brain and strengthening the rest of the retina can reduce the strain on the macula.

I recommend at least five to ten minutes a day of low-stress eye exercises. Start your first week by incorporating palming and thumb rotations into your daily routine. In the second week, try the long swings exercise and the eye scan. These will start to build the resiliency back into your weakened eye, and when you're ready, you can start the 90-day eye protocol below to help reverse your AMD.

(Find the full description of these exercises on my website: https://www.drsamberne.com/eye-exercises/)

DAYS 1-7

- MSM Eye Massage
- Palming
- Thumb Rotations

DAYS 8-14

- Long Swings
- Eye Scan
- Tongue Clock Palming

DAYS 15-21

- Sunning
- Eye Dialogue

DAYS 22-30

- MSM Eye Massage
- Eye Scan

DAYS 31-37

- Sunning
- Eye Dialogue

DAYS 38-46

- MSM Eye Massage
- Eye Scan

DAYS 47-53

- MSM Eye Massage
- Palming
- Thumb Rotations

DAYS 54-60

- Long Swings
- Eye Scan
- Tongue Clock Palming

DAYS 61-69

- MSM Eye Massage
- Eye Scan

DAYS 70-76

- Palming
- Thumb Rotations

DAYS 77-81

- Long Swings
- Eye Scan
- Tongue Clock Palming

DAYS 82-90

- Sunning
- Eye Dialogue
- MSM Eye Massage

CHAPTER 4
MYOPIA & ASTIGMATISM

A healthy eye is shaped like a golf ball. But in several common eye problems, called *refractive errors*, this shape is distorted and results in an inability to correctly focus light – leading to visual distortion. The most common types of refractive errors, myopia and astigmatism, are growing to epidemic proportions.

In the early 2000s, researchers found that 26% of the U.S. population had myopia,[1] and one in three Americans had astigmatism.[2] Experts predict that by 2050, myopia will affect nearly 50% of the world, and it already affects an estimated 4.7 billion people globally.[3]

. . .

These increases are due at least in part to close work with written text and digital devices,[4] and as more children use digital devices for school or learning and adults use them for work, the problem is accelerating!

But there is another, less well-recognized factor leading to myopia and astigmatism: emotion. Remember, the eyes grow out from the brain right as our bodies are forming, and they have a very intimate connection to the mind that goes beyond the ability to see. Both eye and brain tissue are designed to absorb, and just like the brain absorbs visual information, physical stimulation, emotions, and memory, so do the eyes. In other words, when a person takes in visual information through the eyeballs, the data goes through the optic nerve and is processed in the brain. Some visual experiences may stimulate or cause emotions to arise, or even help in holding short and long-term memory. This is why any condition in the eyeball will be reflected throughout your body.

The good news is that, despite what your eye doctor may tell you, your condition is reversible!

WHAT ARE MYOPIA AND ASTIGMATISM?

There is a well-documented connection between these two refractive errors. A study in 2005, for instance, found the presence of astigmatism in children increased the risk factors of an earlier onset of myopia, and severely myopic patients tend to have a high prevalence of astigmatism.[5] However, each condition can also be present independent of the other, and each results from a slightly different distortion in the eye.

Myopia

Myopia, or nearsightedness, occurs in the eye when it becomes slightly elongated from front to back, or when the shape of the cornea or lens is distorted. As a result of its irregular shape, light enters the eye wrong and comes to a focus in front of the retina instead of on it, turning images at a distance blurry. It usually begins in children between six and fourteen, but it can also appear in adults later in life. It tends to worsen with age.

Astigmatism

An eye with astigmatism looks more like an egg than a golf ball. Its irregular shape causes light to enter and focus on two separate points instead of one, causing vision to be distorted both at a distance and close up. Astigmatism starts with an irregular shape in the eyeball that I call a *twist* or *warp*. This twist can cause headaches, eye strain, and anywhere from mild blurring to significant distortion of vision. Astigmatism is most often present at birth, but it can also develop at any time through young adulthood.

WHAT ARE THE CAUSES?

Myopia and astigmatism are most often attributed to genetics, but there is more to the story than that. Think about our ancestors long before these refractive errors became epidemic. They ate more whole plant foods and spent most of their time outside stretching their vision over vast distances, not indoors on glowing digital screens two feet from their eyes. And if we look at the growing deterioration of eye health in more people over time, our ancestors were doing much better.

There are many possible explanations for the increase in myopia and astigmatism: more technology use, greater exposure to environmental toxins, diets too high in highly processed and inflammatory foods.

One of the biggest factors, however, is the increase in work requiring close focus. A study as far back as 1970 among the Inuit people indicated that the introduction of schoolwork into previously unexposed cultures lead to greater instances of myopia,[6] and as recently as 2003, research showed a correlation between increased computer work and myopia in young adults 20 to 30 years old.[7]

This is because myopia is caused usually by a muscle imbalance that gets programmed into our eye system. The tunnel vision of constant close work can be a trigger. Confining our eyes to a field of vision 14 to 20 inches in front of us locks them into a very narrow tunnel of space. As a result, muscle imbalances reshape the eye and distort the vision. When we create such a narrow window of focus, it puts all the stress of vision onto the macula. Over time, this stress becomes a programmed part of the body's response.

Just as any compression in our body extends into our eye tissue, eye stress echoes through our whole system. Our adrenals work extra hard, and epinephrine and cortisol levels go through the roof. This stress response in the body and the visual stress of constant focus up close is the underlying problem that creates a myopic eye.

Astigmatism can be viewed as a twist in the eyeball that's been ingrained into its programming. Just like our myopia reflects in our body, so does astigmatism, and somewhere in the body, a twist is informing the eyes to have astigmatism. Scoliosis, a twist in the hips, can reflect our astigmatic eyes. We can have one leg longer than the other or our hips unaligned. We can have an irregularity in our posture or head position, tilting or leaning to one side or the other. Our neck muscles might be tightly wound. Any impactful twist that occurred in your environment could trigger the onset, even coming out of the birth canal. This twist gets absorbed into the eyes just as it gets absorbed by the brain, developing the body and the eye according to an ingrained internal twist. It not only skews the way you view the world, the twist reflects in your body, your posture and how you carry yourself.

The Eye-Emotion Connection

To dive even deeper, there are emotional causes behind much of the strain in our eye experience.

The bodily stress found in patients with myopia most often results from *fear*. A 2014 study found a correlation between myopia and high stress in childhood.[8] To protect ourselves from whatever it is that makes us feel out of control in our environment, we pull in everything in defense. This hypervigilance keeps the eyes under constant stress. But when you pull the world in, you blur out the distance, reinforcing the tension in your eyes.

The fear behind myopia can cause you to develop strong fixations where you become exclusive in your focus. Your body numbs and you slow or even stop breathing.

As a result, circulation drops, cutting off the eyes and drying them out into a virtual dead zone. The sympathetic nervous system pumps out cortisol. All creativity and decision-making take their information from this defensive "fight-flight-or-freeze" position. This is why distance vision continues to worsen over time.

Astigmatism is both a cause and a result of confusion. Because of their irregular shape and how this affects light entering them, the eyes send conflicting messages to the brain with two different points of focus. An eye doctor usually then reinforces those messages by locking them in place with a corrective lens to cover it up, instead of correcting the muscle imbalance affecting the shape of the eye. A state of confusion can also underlie astigmatism as the result of a cycle of learned and inherited home environmental patterns or a cycle of unhealed trauma that repeats for each generation.

The same emotional message behind our eyes with myopia is often linked to astigmatism, complicating distance sight even further. With astigmatism on top of the blur of myopia, making sense of the world also comes with a twist. Each axis of the warp that astigmatism creates has a meaning and reflects the warp of our inner vision.

• • •

Increased stress driving poor mental health combined with low incidence of treatment can trigger greater family conflict and internalized childhood traumas. In Chinese medicine, psychologically the right eye is the father, and the left, the mother. An infant who grows up watching his parents arguing, or with one parent absent or turned away from the rest of the family, will absorb this imbalance into their left and right eyes. The confusion of an infant witnessing parents in conflict can twist their vision, resulting in astigmatism. The fear of an unsafe home environment can compress the eye with tension, leading to myopia.

WHEN TO SEE A DOCTOR

Most people will notice when their vision at a distance becomes blurry. Up close, your vision may be unaffected; you may even be able to read or see with heightened clarity at very near distances. Across distances, you lose many details. Outlines may seem to disappear, and everything can blur together. If you have trouble reading the scoreboard at a ballgame, you probably have myopia. If you have trouble both at a distance and with reading print that is relatively close to your eyes, you likely have astigmatism.

If you suspect that you have myopia or astigmatism, you should schedule an appointment with an eye doctor. The earlier these conditions are detected, the more effective lifestyle changes will be at reversing them.

Because of the intimate eye-brain connection, there are also visual indicators to detect vision problems in others. Adults can look for signs in children when they may still be too young to notice their own loss of visual acuity. The easiest way to tell is by watching them read and paying attention to movements that indicate a struggle – squinting the eyes, leaning the head, or an overdependence on one eye.

Astigmatism can often precede myopia, and myopia increases the risk of several other eye diseases including macular degeneration, retinal detachment, and glaucoma. So the onset of either should be cause for concern. If your blur is very strong, you may be at risk for other more serious conditions. In addition to causing secondary eye diseases like AMD and glaucoma, a study found that almost 4% of all people diagnosed with nearsightedness actually have a condition called progressive high (or degenerative) myopia (PHM), which occurs at about -6.00 diopters.[9] In addition to the visual blur, PHM comes with other detrimental side effects in the eyes.

Before going further, let's discuss what your prescription actually means. The prescriptions on your myopia lenses are calculated in negative numbers, unlike the drugstore reading glasses for farsighted correction that have a positive symbol. In both cases, the further from zero, the worse the vision. Unlike the rounded shape of the converging lens used for reading, a nearsighted lens is divergent, or concave, because it bends light outward, or diverges it. This makes images that are farther away appear closer and therefore less blurry.

Myopic eyes bring their focus in close so divergent lenses compensate for that focusing power. Without lenses, your eye's focal length is the point where everything becomes blurry, or the "edge of blur." Prescription lenses for myopia diverge the light of images beyond that point to appear much closer and within the eye's range of focus. The correction needed for myopia, measured in negative diopters, represents the inverse of the focal length adjustment in meters. A -2.00 diopter lens, therefore, creates virtual images for the eyes by bending light to make objects appear half a meter away.

If you also have astigmatism, there will be two more numbers. The cylinder describes how flat or irregular your cornea is. The cylinder of astigmatism is also measured in diopters and doctors usually prescribe corrective lenses for anything over 1.5. The last number is the axis, measured in degrees from 0 to 180, and this indicates where on the cornea your astigmatism is located.

The diagnosis you get from your doctor will help you begin to uncover the emotional undercurrent behind your eye-brain-body imbalance. The problem with going to the eye doctor is that they treat the symptoms of blurriness and distortion with a prescription that validates that condition. Prescription lenses do not correct the underlying problems and in fact can make the condition worse! So while I encourage you to visit your eye doctor for an exam to diagnose your myopia and/or astigmatism, take their advice with a grain of salt.

TIPS FOR YOUR EYE EXAM

Here are a few tips for ensuring that you get the most out of your eye appointment.

1. Relax

Going to the doctor is always at least a little stressful, and it can be easy to find yourself at the end of the appointment taking whatever the doctor prescribes as the final word without really understanding it. Furthermore, if your body is constricted from stress or nervousness over the exam, your eyes will be, too, and this will be reflected in how they read the visual acuity eye chart.

You want your eye performing at its best, so remember to blink to keep it moisturized and clean. Eye doctors generally attempt to draw out the maximum prescription in each individual eye, and the resulting lenses program them to become weak. Staying calm will allow your eyes to perform their best, which gives you a clearer baseline of how hard they can still work, and how much they can improve.

2. Go with a friend

A friend can pay attention to the doctor's comments while you might be too hyper-focused on trying to see straight and have trouble remembering later. They can even record audio of the appointment or take notes. While they focus on understanding everything, you can relax during the exam, and then still be able to advocate for yourself with more confidence when it comes down to choosing how you correct your vision after it.

3. Go slow

Breathe deeply while reading and take your time. As part of your exam, the doctor will ask which of two options is clearer to you. If the doctor flips through options one and two so fast that you have no idea which one is better, ask them to slow down and give you a longer view of each. Not only should you take notice of how your eyes feel during the exam, you should stop and feel their connection with the rest of the body. You can even ask your doctor to pause for a minute to do the tongue-clock-hum eye exercise a few times to relax the eyes. Then, come back refreshed and view the chart with improved vision. You end up with a better lens option that can be clear enough, but also relaxing for your eyes.

4. Speak up for yourself

By default, doctors expect you to want them to correct your eyes to 20/20 with lenses, so speak up if that's not what you want. If you have myopia or astigmatism, talk to your doctor about your options. You may want to try a reduced prescription, lenses without astigmatism correction, or separate glasses for distance and computer work. Even if they detect a difference between eyes, request symmetrical lenses that correct both eyes the same so they can start to learn to work together. If you feel comfortable with your current prescription, bring the lenses, and show them to your doctor so they know you want the same or similar. It may not always feel comfortable telling a doctor how to do their job, but their job should also involve taking your needs into consideration.

REDUCE YOUR PRESCRIPTION!

Of course, most doctors will want to correct your vision to 20/20 with lenses. But time and time again, I hear the same story: you go to your eye doctor after getting your prescription lenses complaining of headache, dizziness, and nausea only to get the response, "Don't worry, you'll get used to it." Then, as your eyes get worse, they tell you, "That's just what happens with age. There's nothing you can do about it."

Nearsightedness is not the eyeball's fault – it results from the programming behind the eyeball. When we use lenses, our brain can't process the fear and confusion in our eyes, because our eyes have no idea anything is amiss – the corrective lenses tell them that everything is normal. Once we line up the concepts of normal between our eyes and our brain, we can begin to unravel the programming that told them otherwise.

Except after overcoming my own myopia after living with it for almost 20 years, and helping so many of my patients to do the same, I know this is untrue. With vision therapy, I learned that my nearsightedness was more than in the eyeball. It was in my brain, posture, movement, diet, and emotions. Once I understood what was at the root of my myopia, I knew the steps I needed to take to reverse it. Similarly, in craniosacral therapy, I measure astigmatism in my patients' eyes before the session and then, after I find that twist in their body and unwind it, their measured astigmatism would go away.

. . .

An eyeglass or contact lens prescription is classified as a drug – it's FDA regulated, and only licensed medical professionals can prescribe it. Like any drug, an eye prescription comes with harmful side effects. Though, while doctors will inform you of the potential dangers of a pharmaceutical drug, they never do the same when you start wearing glasses. Instead, they wait until you come back to them complaining of the side effects – dizziness, nausea, neck pain, loss of balance, focus or concentration – and they tell you your body will accommodate the drug: *just get used to it.*

But what happens when you let your body get used to the effects of a drug? It becomes dependent on or, worse, addicted to the prescription. This is what doctors are prescribing when they give the maximum strength and progressively stronger glasses for myopia each year. As a result, the eyes develop a resistance and eventually need more to get the same effect.

Eye prescriptions train the eye and brain to permanently tunnel the vision, putting greater pressure on the macula and more myopia. Add on a strong diopter prescription, and this further compresses and reduces the scale of your vision. The more you wear your prescription, the more this tightens your eyeballs and reinforces the problems that caused your myopia in the first place.

Most prescriptions are already too strong, but this is especially true if you end up using them on your digital devices. Your lens is calculated to work at 20 feet. If you use them for work at 20 inches, you will increase your myopia. Even if you can't switch to a weaker prescription for the parts of your day that require strong distance vision, such as driving, you can definitely get a weaker prescription for using on your computer, phone, or tablet.

A reduced prescription some of the time will help you begin to see the reality of yourself and your life more clearly. The bigger the window of vision, the more relaxed your eyes become, improving depth perception, memory, and information processing. If you currently have two different prescriptions in each eye, balance them out so the eyes can begin to learn to work together. Even with the added blur, weaker, balanced lenses allow the eyes to open up and relax, and the process of adjusting will improve eye flexibility.

Just like the myopia prescription, the corrective astigmatism lens allows the eyes to see clearly, but it covers up the underlying twist in the eyes and body. Wearing astigmatism lenses locks this internal confusion into place and your brain learns to operate under this state as though it were normal. By getting reduced astigmatism or non-astigmatism lenses, you reintroduce your eyes and body to what it feels like to not be in a twisted position.

A minus lens is a potent medicine capable of sharpening your eyesight at a distance, but the side effects come with an emotional cost as well. To get rid of the blur, the corrective lens activates and reprograms the sympathetic branch of the autonomic nervous system that controls eye function, burying the reason your vision blurred in the first place. Prescription lenses cover up the underlying fear and confusion of myopia and astigmatism and give wearers the false sense of security that everything's okay.

Glasses can make people with myopia and astigmatism feel safe. One patient described it this way: "I only know how to control the world when I wear my glasses or contacts." Another said, "I'm addicted to seeing things clearly. I need as many facts as I can get." The part of the mind fixated on survival gets some relief when your eyes process the world through a lens that seems to correct everything, but your inner sight remains unclear. You project your eyesight outside of yourself for it to function correctly. The lens replaces your inner power.

This is why I call myopia an *energy digestion* problem. In patients with myopia, the energy in your eyes is constantly moving outside of them in order to process the energy of the world – there is no receiving. When everything is energy output, not only does seeing become more work, but taking images in becomes much more difficult.

The longer someone has lived with myopic lenses, the more ingrained their fear-based way of seeing. Myopes addicted to the clarity of their prescriptions prefer to avoid taking off their lenses and interacting with their blur, because it's easier than confronting the inner uncertainty that comes with it. But while the myopic bubble can feel safer, reducing myopia is about reducing that external certainty, structure, and density, so the eyes can accept, understand, and begin to heal their blurred reality.

Healing your myopia is about embracing your blur. Blurred vision slows you down and allows you to be more receptive, more psychic, more creative, and better able to go with the flow. When you embrace your blur, you go into your deepest guarded vulnerabilities and the secrets of what caused your nearsightedness. Opening up your tunneled vision and seeing clearly without lenses or a reduced prescription is a byproduct of taking full responsibility and loving your blur.

. . .

Of course, any changes you make to your prescription will result in some decrease in visual clarity. There will be some blur, so only incorporate the reduced lenses for use during low or zero-demand situations. Try to start taking off your glasses for a minimum of 30 minutes a day, and very quickly you'll feel how much stress they're putting onto your eyes. Remember, you don't want to stress the eyes out even more, so if you're squinting or straining to see, put the glasses back on.

While it may be my number one recommendation for reducing myopia and astigmatism, a reduced prescription will only be effective once you've developed a deeper trust with your eyes. A mind that has been programmed for so long into one way of interpreting the world will become overwhelmed and reject the reduced prescription without doing this work first. Start with the eye exercises recommended below to begin the process of relaxing your eyes, and then you can make the transition into a 30% reduced lens.

When you make a daily practice out of retraining your eyes, the eyeball will return to its spherical shape, no longer needing astigmatism correction, and the tension in the eyes will dissolve, eliminating the myopia.

OTHER RECOMMENDATIONS

In addition to reducing your prescription, there are a number of other steps you can take that will improve your vision.

Diet

Like any kind of eye deterioration, myopia and astigmatism can also be compounded by poor eye nutrition. Myopia and astigmatism put a lot of stress on the retina, which has one of the highest metabolic needs in the body. A lack of nourishment to the eyes can interrupt the metabolic systems needed to successfully restore their health.

Trace Minerals

Particularly for the progressive pattern of myopia, the trace mineral chromium can help in slowing things down. Research suggests that people with myopia tend to be deficient in this nutrient.[10] The body uses chromium to help break down foods and regulate blood sugar. Low chromium levels can impair glucose metabolism in the eyes, causing fluids to build up and create pressure, increasing myopia.

. . .

Oats, barley, broccoli, and sweet potato are great sources of chromium to add to your diet. While food sources of chromium are abundant, the absorption rate into the body is low. Adults should consume between 25 and 35 micrograms of chromium per day, and consuming it with vitamin C helps to boost its low dietary absorption rate.[11]

Selenium and magnesium are also important trace minerals for eye health. Research suggests selenium may be helpful in treating thyroid eye disease, which can include swelling of the soft tissue around the eyes,[12] a reaction which may also aid in relaxing the tension of myopia. Magnesium improves blood flow to the eye and a 2014 study found it to be promising in the management of glaucoma, which is a condition of high intraocular pressure and linked to myopia.[13]

Healthy Oils

As we've seen, omega-3s are critical for eye health. Concentration of the omega-3 called DHA is particularly high in the retina. Research has found omega-3s to have protective effects in the retina, and some studies have shown that consumption of omega-3s is linked with decreased dry eye disease.[14] A 2012 study found that DHA supplementation could block a toxin build-up in the retina of mice, implicating a role in the prevention of age-related vision deterioration.[15]

While most people have no problem finding enough omega-6 in sources like their common cooking oils, omega-3s are more valuable for improving cardiovascular health and eye function. Adults should consume between 1000 and 2000 milligrams of omega-3s per day. You can add these into your diet by eating more salmon, herring, or sardines, or you can supplement with fish or algae oil.

Promote Overall Nutrition

Of course, all other dietary recommendations for optimal eye health will help your eyes to function properly so they can release their pent-up tension and relax their twisted form. Focus on a diet high in plant foods with colors that span the rainbow. Cut out inflammatory foods like processed carbohydrates and sugars.

Add eye-healthy herbs to your diet. Cilantro is a carotenoid plant with potent antioxidant qualities and anti-inflammatory effects. Animal studies suggest it may be useful in managing diabetes and hyperglycemia.[16] Cilantro also contains eye-healthy vitamins and minerals like magnesium and vitamins A, B2 and C. Fresh basil may help bring down high blood pressure,[17] contains eye-healthy vitamins and minerals, like magnesium and vitamin A, as well as the antioxidants lutein, zeaxanthin, and beta-carotene to help fight free radicals and cell damage in the eyes. Cinnamon lowers blood glucose levels,[18] improves brain function,[19] helps the digestive system function more effectively, and is one of the most antioxidant-rich foods in the world.[20]

The master antioxidant, glutathione, is critical to improve oxygenation and hydration in the eye, eliminating free radicals and clearing the buildup of metabolic waste. Improving metabolic processes releases the buildup of pressure in the eye. Asparagus is the best plant-based source of glutathione. Sulfur-based foods like garlic, shallots, and cruciferous vegetables will also help boost glutathione levels.

Open Your Vision and Your Mind

To embrace the blur and the emotions behind our myopia and astigmatism, we need to uncover the history that locked those emotions into place. By changing the way we use our physical eyes, we can open up our eyes and minds to a new way of understanding vision. Learn to open up your eyes and your mind in order to release the underlying emotions trapped inside of these narrowed visual windows.

• • •

The tunneled vision of myopia wants our focus to stay narrow, so try to see the "big view" by opening up your peripheral vision and taking in the whole environment around you. This helps to reduce pressure on the macula. Strong peripheral vision gives us improved depth perception, balance, and orientation, and facilitates cognitive processing, including memory.

Myopia wants us to see only down and in, so make a practice of looking up and out into the distance. If your work keeps you focused 20 inches in front of you, commit to the 20/20/20 rule: look 20 feet away from you, every 20 minutes for about 20 seconds. This will prevent the accumulation of visual stress and support flexibility in the eyes.

Another way to open your vision is to go outside and be in nature. You will feel the impact on your brain and body. Not only will you relax your mind and muscles, spending time outdoors will boost your vitamin D levels, encourage more exercise, elevate your mood, improve concentration, and help your body speed up its healing process.[21]

• • •

Being outside is also great for expanding your vision and relieving stress in the eyes.

With our electronics and technology increasingly keeping us spending more time indoors, many of us are suffering from what has been termed Nature Deficit Disorder. Since author Richard Louv coined the unofficial diagnosis of Nature Deficit Disorder in 2006, thousands of studies have connected an increasing withdrawal from nature with "diminished use of the senses, attention difficulties, conditions of obesity and higher rates of emotional and physical illness."[22] Children who spend more time outside have been found to be less likely to develop myopia.[23] For maximum benefits, spend at least 30 minutes a day outside in the sun.

Find Holistic Practitioners

It's important to find a primary eye health professional who will focus on healing your myopia and astigmatism instead of covering them up. Look for a professional who advocates for a cause-based approach.

Expand your own methods of managing eye health beyond the primary eye doctor. Seek out body workers, craniosacral therapists, or Rolfers who can begin to unwind your eyes and body from the astigmatism.

• • •

I recommend going straight into eliminating the astigmatism correction in your lenses. If you leave the eye prescription the same while doing body work, you untwist the body, but the eye muscles cannot release. But the combination of a reduce prescription with body work will strengthen and straighten both the eye and the body. Invariably, after an hour-long session of craniosacral therapy, my patients' prescription on the eye chart will come out at about 30% less than measured before the session.

Blue Light Blockers

The amount of work people do on their computers, phones, and tablets has caused enough digital eye strain for the American Optometric Association to coin the condition as "computer vision syndrome."[24] As work and entertainment increasingly go online, it will become harder to expect anyone to be able to decrease their screen time, but we can better protect our eyes during it. Considering the links between close-work and myopia and blue light and stress on the eyes, it's safe to say that blue-light blockers can assist in healing your vision.

Blue light is a chaotic wave frequency in a very short form, and while not all blue light is bad for your eyes, when it falls between 400 and 460 nanometers, this light can be highly damaging. A 2019 study by the French government found excessive blue light exposure affected eye and retinal health and accelerated the progression of AMD and dry eye. They found blue light, at minimum, to cause eye strain and fatigue, and after 6:00PM, it suppresses melatonin production, which can disrupt your sleep.

Choose a blue-blocking option that deflects the highest amount of blue light possible. You can get blue-light filters embedded into glasses or buy a blocking tint to go over your lenses or screens. Some of my patients complain that the tints make the screen appear too dark. They can also create an imbalance of color getting into the eyes, which can dilate the pupil more and let more of the harmful light in than they block out. I find the filters to offer the best protection without adding any tint that can affect color imbalance and pupil size.

Eye Drops

Screen time affects our ability to produce tears, so eye drops can help keep our eyes moist and healthier, but remember, not all eye drops are created equal. Most you can find in the pharmacy are full of chemical preservatives and end up drying your eyes even more. Pharmaceutical drops may offer some help with the symptoms, but come with other side effects. Go for natural MSM or homeopathic eye drops, and follow these tips when applying:

1. Wash your hands first.
2. Don't put them directly into your eye. Lay with your head back and run drops along your eyelashes and open your eyes to give them an eye bath. Use six to eight drops, all at once or massaged in individually onto your eyelids and eyelashes. Do this four to eight times a day, every hour or two.
3. Give yourself a hexane-free organic castor oil massage before bed. This helps your eyes keep from getting dry overnight when they are most prone to it.
4. Use herbal compresses of red raspberry leaf tea, eyebright, or goldenseal.

WHAT ABOUT SURGERY?

Just like prescription lenses, surgery addresses the symptoms, but never the cause that led those symptoms to develop. This means the causes still exist and will likely return if never addressed. Often, you will hear about people getting LASIK surgery for nearsightedness – only to find out that, after a few years of corrected vision, their vision once again starts to deteriorate.

LASIK or implanted contact lenses are external solutions, and they can't solve an internal problem. You may have some mild success with implanted lenses over LASIK, especially in cases of moderate to high myopia, but still with side effects – eye strain, red eyes, double vision, glaucoma, and cataracts. This is because healing the eyes needs to come from the inside out.

EYE EXERCISES FOR ASTIGMATISM AND MYOPIA

I recommend the above changes in combination with a daily exercise program. Instead of treating the symptoms and driving the underlying cause further in, this holistic approach helps you identify that underlying problem causing your myopia or astigmatism. This way your symptoms, and the condition, can go away for good.

Adding a few minutes of any vision therapy exercises at any point in your day will work to recharge and replenish your eyes. If you work on a computer all day, interrupt that pattern at regular intervals with these exercises to improve eye resilience. Add an exercise break at least every two hours so your eyes can regenerate from the debilitating effects of screen time.

When you feel ready to incorporate the full routine, below is my 90-day eye exercise protocol for reducing myopia and astigmatism. Follow this and your eyes will soon work more effectively with a lower or non-astigmatism lens and the blur will start to clear up. By the end of 90 days, if you've incorporated as many of these recommendations into your day as possible, you won't need glasses at all because you will have healed your eyes.

(Find the full description of these exercises on my website: https://www.drsamberne.com/eye-exercises/)

Days 1-7

- Figure 8 Eye Massage
- N Breath and Palm Hum
- Eye Dialogue
- Plus Lens to Blur

Days 8-14

- Sunning
- Tongue Clock Palming
- Plus Lens to Blur

Days 15-21

- Long Swings
- Yin Yang Chart (no glasses)
- Eye Brain Body Fun
- Plus Lens to Blur

Days 22-30

- Figure 8 Eye Massage
- The Thumb Game
- Plus Lens to Blur

Days 31-37

- Sunning
- N Breath and Palm Hum
- Eye Dialogue

Days 38-46

- Yin Yang Chart
- Figure 8 Eye Massage
- Tongue Clock

DR. SAM BERNE

Days 47-53

- Sunning
- MSM Eye Massage
- Eye Brain Body Fun

DAYS 54-60

- Long Swings
- The Thumb Game
- N Breath and Palm Hum

DAYS 61-69

- Eye Scan
- Yin Yang Chart
- Figure 8 Eye Massage
- Plus Lens to Blur

DAYS 70-76

- Eye Dialogue
- The Thumb Game
- Tongue Clock Palming

DAYS 77-81

- Long Swings
- The Thumb Game
- Yin Yang Chart
- Plus Lens to Blur

DAYS 82-90

- N Breath and Palm Hum
- Eye Brain Body Fun
- Figure 8 Eye Massage

CHAPTER 5
HYPEROPIA & PRESBYOPIA

If you've reached your 40s or 50s, chances are good that at some point you have found yourself pushing your reading material away from your face in order to see it more clearly. In this classic sign of aging, your eyes have begun to lose their ability to focus close up.

Several different conditions can cause this loss of near vision, collectively called "farsightedness." The two most common conditions are refractive errors called hyperopia and presbyopia. Presbyopia is a more advanced form of hyperopia that increases with age. Just like with myopia, there are both physical and emotional causes that underlie these two conditions. And just like with myopia, you can heal your condition with a combination of therapy, diet, and exercise.

WHAT ARE HYPEROPIA AND PRESBYOPIA?

If objects close to your face are blurry and you find yourself squinting to see clearly while reading, writing, or other close work, you may have hyperopia or presbyopia. Other symptoms may include eye strain, burning, aches or discomfort in or around the eyes, or headaches, especially when focusing the eyes close up. These symptoms may feel more pronounced when you're tired or in dim lighting.

Hyperopia

Hyperopia, or farsightedness, is a refractive error that is in many ways opposite of myopia. Where myopia indicates an elongated shape of the eye causing the image to focus in front of the retina, hyperopia indicates an eye that is too short, and images focus behind the retina. As a result, images that are closer to your face will appear blurry, whereas at a distance your vision may remain sharp.

According to NEI's 2019 statistical data, there are over 14 million cases of hyperopia in the U.S. alone.[1] The most common form this condition takes is simple hyperopia, where the eye has a decreased axial length from a flattened cornea, thickened lens, or other damage affecting their curvature. Atypical development, trauma, or disease of the eye such as cataracts can cause hyperopia, but this form is less common. Because the eyeball is misshapen, muscle imbalances develop.

While myopic eyes can see at close distances, hyperopic eyes see objects at greater distances more clearly than they do up close. The degree of hyperopia will affect your degree of symptoms, which can range from mild to severe. In some mild cases, people may not yet notice any blur, but with moderate hyperopia you will likely start noticing a loss of focus on nearby objects. In severe cases, both near and far distances may be blurred.

There are different ranges of hyperopia can be divided according to the diopter (the unit of measure for prescriptions) strength:

- Low hyperopia: +2.00 or less
- Moderate hyperopia: +2.25 to +5.00
- High or Severe Hyperopia: +5.25

Most cases are mild enough to correct with drugstore reading glasses and most people only use them on occasions where they work up close. However, some people may have such severe hyperopia that it affects their vision near, far, and all the time.

Presbyopia

Presbyopia is a more advanced form of hyperopia. As the hyperopic eye ages, muscle imbalances worsen. The ciliary muscles that surround the lens of the eye are responsible for reshaping it in order to focus, a process known as *accommodation*. For distance, the muscles relax, but for objects up close, they contract to curve the lens and change its focusing power. If these ciliary muscles weaken, or if the lens becomes harder to flex, the eyes lose their ability to focus. These imbalances usually occur in adults over 40.

WHAT ARE THE CAUSES?

Hyperopia

Most infants are actually born with a mild degree of hyperopia, but as the eyeball lengthens and grows to its full size, it learns to focus properly, and the condition lessens. Since children's eyes have a stronger ability to accommodate, they can experience up to moderate amounts of hyperopia without any noticeable blur.

By the age of six to nine months, the prevalence of hyperopia decreases to less than 9%. By the time they reach the age of one, less than 4% of children still have the condition. Since it can emerge in adulthood as accommodation decreases, the rates jump back up to 9.9% by age 40.[2] One study found that 62% of adults over 40 develop hyperopia.[3]

In addition to age, a number of other factors increase the likelihood of developing hyperopia. If you have a first-degree family member with the condition, your chances increase, suggesting a genetic component. A 2011 study linked a higher risk of hyperopia with cases of maternal smoking during pregnancy.[4] One study in India found the incidence of refractive error, including hyperopia, to be more prevalent in urban areas rather than rural ones.[5] Many genetic conditions include hyperopia as symptoms, including:

- microphthalmia
- achromatopsia
- aniridia
- Leber congenital amaurosis
- X-linked juvenile retinoschisis
- Senior-Løken syndrome
- Gorlin-Chaudhry-Moss syndrome
- Down syndrome
- fragile X syndrome[6]

Presbyopia

Most doctors attribute the sole cause of presbyopia to old age. The word itself comes from the Greek "presbys," meaning *older person* and "opsis," meaning *vision* or *eye*. This is because our natural eye lenses are soft and flexible as children, but with age, they tend to harden and become rigid, resulting in blurry vision up close. But laying all the blame on age ignores all of the preventable damage that happens along the way.

While the obvious factor in developing presbyopia is age, only some people's near vision deteriorates with age. Medical conditions like diabetes, multiple sclerosis, or cardiovascular disease can lead to a premature onset of presbyopia in adults under 40 and pharmaceutical drugs, like antidepressants, antihistamines, and diuretics can also accelerate the process.[7]

One of the main causes for the rapid growth in cases of presbyopia is our excessive **digital device use**. Focus for long periods of time at one distance hardens the lens and reduces muscle flexibility. If we're wearing progressive or multifocal lenses while we do our computer work, this puts even more stress on our eyes and brain to make seeing possible. Through these lenses, we narrow our focus even more to fit through even tinier windows in our focusing system, increasing visual stress and accelerating the presbyopia.

People often make the mistake of using the same corrective lens for multiple distances, including when they work on a computer. Using a lens that corrects at 10 to 15 inches for distances over 20 will accelerate the deterioration of your eyes. This is why you should also always take your magnifiers off when you look across the room, or your eyes may also begin to deteriorate for distance.

Oxidative stress can also accelerate presbyopia. When you're not getting enough oxygenation and hydration into the eye tissue, especially the lens, this causes waste to accumulate, further dehydrating the eye and blocking the vital nutrients that could repair it.

Monovision corrective lenses, where one eye is corrected for distance or one eye is corrected for near, puts incredible stress on the near eye to do all the focusing. Doctors may prescribe monovision corrections through LASIK or cataract surgery, but I never recommend getting them. Particularly in concurrent cases with presbyopia, this will accelerate the deterioration of your near vision.

• • •

Another big risk is using **magnification lenses**. I know what you're thinking: "But that's what they give us to correct our farsightedness!" *Exactly*. Those very same reading magnifiers are the reason your eyes continue to have blurred near vision and what keeps that vision deteriorating further. Especially when you use them while doing computer work, this will put excess stress on your eye muscles by making them work harder.

One of the tests I do with my patients allows me to tell if both eyes are focusing on the same task or if the brain is suppressing or shutting off one of their eyes, and I've seen patients with presbyopia not using both of their eyes together. One eye tends to do all of the work, but gets more fatigued, resulting in a weakened focusing ability. The magnification lenses, on or off the computer, will make the one working eye do even more work, causing more stress and more rapid deterioration.

The Eye-Emotion Connection

As with myopia and astigmatism, there can be emotional causes that underlie hyperopia and presbyopia.

Farsightedness and nearsightedness are opposite adaptive responses to the external world. With nearsightedness, the primary emotion is fear, and our minds are stuck in the past. We pull the world closer to compensate. The emotion behind farsightedness, on the other hand, is anger. The mind is always looking to the future, and the behavioral compensation is to push the world away. In Asian medicine, the major organ associated with anger is the liver – the organ with energy meridians that most influence eye health.

With all farsightedness, the programming behind our eyes is pushing the world away from us, just like we hold the newspaper out farther away from our face in order to read it. We want the world to be bigger and see a broader picture, but our arms are never long enough. You'll first notice the onset of presbyopia as blurred vision at a normal reading distance, and you'll instinctively push it away to try and focus. Either from weakened ciliary muscles or a hardened lens, your eyes have lost the ability to accommodate without magnifying glasses.

We already know that any weakness or imbalance in the eye is reflected in the body, and farsighted behaviors will also show up in our movement and posture, our thoughts, preferences, and emotional reactions. Farsightedness is a type of mental flaccidity and aversion to detail. Whereas nearsighted people have mastered the details but struggle to see the whole picture, in farsightedness, the details can be stressful. The metaphor for farsightedness is, "I'm a global person who can see the whole picture, but it's hard for me to manifest my vision into detail and steps towards taking action."

WHEN TO SEE A DOCTOR

While most cases of hyperopia and presbyopia are mild, the condition can negatively impact on your quality of life. If you're having trouble with your near vision to the point that you have trouble with reading or other necessary tasks, or if it takes away from your enjoyment of activities, it's time for a visit to the doctor.

Proper treatment is essential to prevent complications from your condition. Unaddressed hyperopia can lead to the development of other eye conditions, including strabismus (crossed eyes) or amblyopia (lazy eye). Levels greater than +1.00 refractive difference between eyes, or hyperopic eyes over +5.00, can induce amblyopia. Infants with uncorrected hyperopia over +3.50 are up to 13 times more likely to develop strabismus.[8] Research has also linked uncorrected hyperopia with impaired literacy standards in children,[9] which is why early detection is critical to ensure healthy learning and development. Farsightedness can also impair your safety. A 2019 study found that uncorrected hyperopia can increase the risk of falls even when eyes show normal acuity, suggesting a link between the condition and balance.[10]

Strabismus, anisometropia, or a binocular or accommodative dysfunction may be indicative of a concurrent hyperopia that is not yet manifesting symptoms, so check with your eye doctor if you have any of these other eye conditions.

Other conditions may mimic the symptoms of farsightedness, which is why it's important to get an accurate diagnosis. Visual stress, hypoglycemia, cataracts and post-refractive surgery, orbital tumors, a serious elevation of the retina, and posterior scleritis may also cause difficulty with near vision. But as they result from different causes, they will require different treatments.

A Word of Caution About Doctors

Most prescribed treatments for farsightedness can actually worsen your problem – so it's important to be sure you see the right practitioner.

This is especially true for children whose eyes are still developing. When a child visits the doctor, most will dilate the pupils before they take their visual acuity exam. This paralyzes the muscles to their weakest and results in the strongest possible corrective prescription. These lenses then artificially preserve the maximum visual acuity in the child's eyes, stunting their natural function and growth. Even I learned this method of measuring acuity, but these lenses are too strong and distorting, especially for a child still undergoing transformations in organic visual development.

What most eye doctors measure is "sight," or the ability to see a letter at 20 feet, but this isn't vision. Vision is a developmentally-learned skill involving the eyes, brain, and body working together. Many vision problems in the eyes are due to an interference in sensory-motor delays, toxicities, stress, and birth traumas. These experiences can occur before we learn to speak, even sometimes in-utero.

Instead of just going to any eye doctor, look for someone who can provide a developmental vision evaluation that not only measures sight, refraction for glasses, and eye health, but also the developmental motor skills, including the primitive reflexes, vestibular resiliency, and bilateral motor skills. They should also assess more specific visual skills like tracking, focusing, coordination, and perceptual skills like memory, figure ground, and other cognitive processing skills.

Similarly, visiting your doctor with symptoms of presbyopia will result in them telling you that your loss of near vision acuity will worsen until you're 65 and nothing can be done to stop it. They'll prescribe you the maximum plus lens diopter strength to magnify your focusing power on near objects and say that's all they can do.

The problem with this as their one and only solution is that magnifiers make the eyes worse. Reading magnifiers eliminate the eye's practice of focusing on detail while seeing the whole picture because they distort the images into something much bigger than they really are. They relax the ciliary muscles to the point that they atrophy from lack of use. Magnifiers disconnect you from your focusing muscles, and so you need more and more magnification to make the same correction. Eventually, you progress to wearing a bifocal and then you need your farsighted glasses all the time.

WHAT CAN I DO ABOUT IT?

Remember, your diagnosis is not a life sentence! While common wisdom says farsightedness is incurable and vision loss is inevitable with old age, I believe that vision therapy can not only slow down, but even reverse the progression of both hyperopia and presbyopia.

Rethink Your Corrective Lenses

Most often, a doctor will prescribe magnifying lenses for either type of farsightedness. Unlike myopic lenses, the magnifiers are convex, or rounded, which bends the light rays to compensate for the shortened eye, so they land on the retina instead of behind it. But just like the prescriptions for myopia and astigmatism, these lenses are drugs. Your magnifiers correct the blur but come with side effects, including visual stress and the paralyzing and reducing of the ciliary muscles' resiliency. Eventually, like a drug, you become dependent on them.

A farsighted lens makes the world artificially larger than it really is, which decreases eye muscle responsiveness and pushes them towards flaccidity. This is why your magnification needs to increase every time you go to the eye doctor until the problem gets so bad it also affects your distance vision. The doctor may then upgrade the prescription to a bifocal, or even trifocal, but multifocal lenses force your eyes to split the world into small areas, making it even harder for them to focus.

If you already have multifocal lenses, remember only to wear them in circumstances where you need to shift your focus back and forth between near and far. Never use them for extended periods of time or during activities that need concentrated focus like driving, reading, or using a computer. Instead, a single vision lens will help your eyes access much more of their peripheral vision, supporting better depth perception, visual memory, and body balance skills.

If I discovered a child's eyes to be hyperopic, I would hesitate to prescribe any kind of corrective lens, especially if they have no symptoms. Their visual system still has a lot of ability to grow and change, meaning physical eye therapy exercises can be very effective. Giving a child the maximum prescription and making them wear it full-time only reinforces the farsightedness and makes it harder to reverse.

I might consider a minimal diopter lens at half the strength based on the child's focusing response while reading, but both eyes would be balanced despite any difference in acuity measurements to encourage them to work together. In combination with a reduced prescription, I would take the child through a whole-body physical eye therapy program and cognitive visual processing in perception. This will integrate their primitive reflexes to improve their balance, vestibular system, and vision as well as bilateral interaction between the eyes, brain, and body. If a child can learn to focus their body through space, the farsightedness in the eyes starts to reduce.

For farsighted adults, on the other hand, can be harder nuts to crack. Despite its Greek name, presbyopia is less about the number of years you've lived and more about the two eyes not working together. The problem is that by 40, our eyes and brain have already learned quite a bit about how things work, and it can be harder to change our minds. It will take a complete reeducation of the eye's muscular flexibility to wean you off the need for the magnification lens, which is why vision therapy is the only practice that can interrupt our visual patterns and replace them with new ones.

If you're an adult with hyperopia or presbyopia, your magnifiers are probably too strong. Go to the drugstore with a book or your laptop and try on different diopter strengths until you find the lowest possible magnification lens that provides both clarity and comfort at 14 inches. For example, if you can read print books at +1.50, you can use even less for the computer screen because it's usually another eight to 10 inches away. You can also expand the size of on-screen fonts and get an even lower prescription.

Pinhole Glasses

Another option that corrects your farsighted vision without a prescription or side effects are pinhole glasses. These look like regular glasses, except instead of clear glass lenses, your eyes look through blackened windows filled with tiny holes. You can use them to read fine print or do close work, but they're not practical for full time wear. Normally, the pupil regulates how much light gets into the eye, bundling the diverging light rays from an object into a single "pencil of light," which is where a refractive error usually occurs. With pinhole glasses, the tiny holes narrow that pencil by limiting the peripheral light that enters the eye, diminishing the refractive error and allowing the eye to focus more clearly.

Instead of disconnecting you from your eye muscles like magnifiers, pinhole glasses teach you to focus them in a more concentrated way. You can also use them to exercise your eyes. Try putting them on and reading for one-minute intervals, taking them off for a rest in between. Be mindful of what your eyes and brain are experiencing in order to see detail again. Are your eyes moving more? Are you breathing more? Is your body relaxing more? Developing this awareness will help you understand what you need to focus on better.

Gabor Patch

A Gabor patch is a type of visual stimulation in a controlled environment that is designed to improve contrast sensitivity and processing speed. You look at black and white parallel lines oriented at different angles and with varying levels of clarity and size that are flashed in patterns at different speeds to stimulate the visual cortex.

I tried this eye exercise program for a week myself, and my visual recognition and reaction time increased, but there were some major flaws.

One big problem with Gabor patches is that they invite no conversation between the exercises and the eyes themselves.

Further, considering this is a program on a digital device, I was also struck by how they made no recommendations to use blue-light protection, which is one of the main drivers of near vision deterioration. I recommend physical therapy eye exercises in free spaces without technology, since returning to a more natural experience allows you to work with your visual system in its natural environment.

If you want to try out a Gabor patch program, I recommend two additions:

- Incorporate eye exercises to improve muscle flexibility and visual coordination
- Use blue-blocking filters

Diet

As always, stick to an eye-healthy diet to accompany your regimen of eye exercises and lifestyle changes. The simple action of adding more plants to your daily menu gives you a boost of antioxidants, eye nutrients and fiber for a healthy gut. Eat more nutrient-dense foods for eye health like bilberry and asparagus. Flavonoids are critical for reducing UV-induced oxidative stress, and quercetin is a common flavanol with potent antioxidant effects. Studies have found quercetin to be effective in reducing oxidative stress and inflammatory biomarkers.[11]

Chapter 8 contains a more complete description on the dietary connection between these nutrients and our eyes. But there are some specific nutritional recommendations for improving your farsightedness.

Include:

- Vitamins A, B-complex, C, and E
- Lutein, zeaxanthin, and astaxanthin
- Trace minerals like magnesium, selenium, and chromium for muscular flexibility
- Glutathione, the "master antioxidant"
- Omega-3s

Avoid:

- Caffeine
- Gluten
- Dairy
- Sugar
- Processed foods
- Trans fats

Eye Drops

Keep your natural eye lenses soft and flexible by hydrating them more. Start with the 5% MSM drop and apply four to six times a day, or whenever your eyes feel dry.

Blue Blockers

I've already mentioned the blue blockers for those of you interested in trying the Gabor patch program, but I would also recommend these for anyone who has a lot of screen time during the day. Protect your eyes from the oxidative stress that can cause your vision loss by reducing the visual stressors on your eyes wherever you can.

WHAT ABOUT SURGERY?

By now, you should know that I think eye surgery should only be used as a last resort, and that lifestyle changes and eye exercises can be a more effective and longer-lasting treatment method without the harmful side effects. However, it may be useful to know about some common surgery options for hyperopia and presbyopia.

Conductive Keratoplasty

Using radiofrequency energy, doctors performing this surgery will direct heat around the cornea to diminish its edges and enhance its curve, which results in an improved ability to focus. However, results vary in effectiveness, and they may not last long.[12]

Refractive Lens Exchange

Similar to cataract surgery, this process removes the natural lens and implants an artificial one to correct the hyperopia. This can be good for high level cases, but reading glasses may still be necessary after the procedure. It also carries the same risks as cataract surgery – inflammation, infection, bleeding, and glaucoma.[13]

LASIK Surgery

One of the most popular options for vision correction, this surgery gives the cornea a more pronounced dome-shape to adjust its focusing, but it can only correct near vision up to +5.00.

Even if your farsightedness falls under that range, refractive surgery only changes the prescription in the eyeball, not the programming behind the eye. Our posture, movement habits, early childhood, diet, stress, birth, trauma, and toxicity, especially over long periods of time, all play a role in programming our eyes. When the time comes for refractive surgery that only corrects the eyeball, Which do you think ends up being longer lasting: the surgery or the programming? The programming, every time.

That is why refractive surgery never lasts. Over time, the prescription begins to creep back into the eyes. Surgery fixed the eyeball problem, but the problem still exists in the brain, leaving you forever questioning your vision. You can't trust it because of the mismatch between the body prescription and the eye prescription. Physical eye therapy, on the other hand, through its re-education process, can bridge the gap between the two and eventually create eye-brain-body unity.

Corneal Inlays

One of the newer eye surgeries offered for farsightedness, doctors implant these tiny devices into the cornea of the non-dominant eye to restore close vision by increasing its depth of focus. This can be a refractive corneal inlay or small aperture inlay, which inserts a ring with a pinhole opening at the center that focuses light in the same way as pinhole glasses. This procedure is not recommended for people with other refractive errors, corneal diseases, cataracts, or dry eye conditions, and some people may have a cornea that is too thick for this surgery. Side effects include glare, halos, poor night vision or difficulty reading in dim light. Complications can include scarring, swelling, inflammation, and corneal thinning or clouding.[14]

Refractive Surgery for Monovision

I've already warned about the dangers of monovision, but it is a common recommendation for doctors to give to patients looking for an alternative to magnifiers. Using a laser, the surgeon reshapes the cornea in the dominant eye to correct for distance visual acuity and does the same but for close-up vision in the other. Many people find it difficult to adapt to this corrective approach and you should definitely try monovision corrective lenses before jumping right into surgery. Side effects include the loss of depth perception, and you may still end up needing to use magnifiers anyway in certain cases like reading fine print.[15]

EYE EXERCISES FOR FARSIGHTEDNESS

Instead of surgeries that confuse your eye-brain connection, or corrective lenses that deteriorate your near vision even further, I recommend a combination of lifestyle changes and eye exercises to correct your vision more permanently. Even if you already wear reading glasses, these exercises will help reverse the atrophy and increase flexibility in your ciliary muscles so that you don't need them anymore.

Changing vision is a process, not an overnight success, but if you're diligent and disciplined, you'll start to wean yourself off the powerful plus lenses. When you're ready and disciplined enough to stick with it, you can start my 90-day eye exercise protocol for reducing farsightedness and begin the process of healing your vision.

(Find the full description of these exercises on my website: https://www.drsamberne.com/eye-exercises/)

DAYS 1-7

- Figure 8 Eye Massage
- N Breath and Palm Hum

VITAL VISION

- Eye Dialogue

DAYS 8-14

- Sunning
- Tongue Clock Palming

DAY 15-21

- Long Swings
- Yin Yang Chart (no glasses)
- Eye Brain Body Fun

141

DR. SAM BERNE

DAYS 22-30

- Figure 8 Eye Massage
- The Thumb Game

DAYS 31-37

- Sunning
- N Breath and Palm Hum
- Eye Dialogue

DAYS 38-46

- Yin Yang Chart
- Figure 8 Eye Massage
- Tongue Clock

DAYS 47-53

- Sunning
- MSM Eye Massage
- Eye Brain Body Fun

DAYS 54-60

- Long Swings
- The Thumb Game
- N Breath and Palm Hum

DAYS 61-69

- Eye Scan
- Yin Yang Chart
- Figure 8 Eye Massage

DAYS 70-76

- Eye Dialogue
- The Thumb Game
- Tongue Clock Palming

DAYS 77-81

- Long Swings
- The Thumb Game
- Yin Yang Chart

DR. SAM BERNE

DAYS 82-90

- N Breath and Palm Hum
- Eye Brain Body Fun
- Figure 8 Eye Massage

CHAPTER 6
STRABISMUS, AMBLYOPIA, AND DIPLOPIA

Diplopia (double vision) and amblyopia (known as lazy eye) are vision problems that involve the two eyes being misaligned with one another. However, they are much more than just eye problems: They are a symptom of an integration problem between the brain and body.

Since they both involve an eye-brain misconnection, addressing these conditions in a holistic way often involves an overlap. Both amblyopia and diplopia are often caused by strabismus, or crossed eyes, in which one eye fails to line up properly with the other. Children are born with strabismus in fifty percent of known cases,[1] and without early detection it can lead to lazy eye or double vision. These eye problems could also be covering up a more serious condition in the brain.

. . .

Although early detection is important, doctors often wrongly assume that surgery early in life is the only treatment for these conditions, and that the misalignment will be permanent if not addressed in childhood. This could not be farther from the truth! My success in helping people reduce double vision is to treat the whole person, not just the eye muscles. The secret to success is to show the person how the brain is the traffic director in learning how to direct the eye muscles. This occurs through a sequential application of physical eye therapy that includes primitive reflex therapy, gross and fine motor exercises, vestibular therapy, craniosacral therapy, and nutritional guidance.

The standard treatments for these conditions are ineffective because they only treat the symptoms, not the cause. To really reverse the condition and get both eyes and the brain all communicating together again, you must rethink how you imagine the muscles of the eye, their connection with the brain and body, and how they all need to work together towards recovery.

WHAT ARE STRABISMUS, AMBLYOPIA, AND DIPLOPIA?

Strabismus

A patient with strabismus has one eye that does not point in the same direction as the other. If the person is looking up, one eye may fail to move in alignment with the other and may point inward, for instance. The eyes can cross inward or outward or have a vertical deviation. Because of the eye-brain misfire, there's usually a lack of body integration along with strabismus, especially in kids with developmental delays.

In some cases, the weaker eye is always out of alignment, but in others, the problem comes and goes intermittently. *Strabismus does not, on its own, impair a person's eyesight*, but it does cause difficulty in the brain's ability to interpret images – especially in intermittent cases. Symptoms include poor depth perception, eye strain, and headaches.

Amblyopia

Amblyopia, on the other hand, *is* a visual impairment. It is caused by one eye being significantly weaker than the other. In kids, you may notice poor depth perception or indications of a visual struggle, like squinting, shutting one eye, or tilting the head when trying to focus.

Lazy eye often goes undetected until a child's first eye exam. The symptoms with lazy eye can be hard to detect because the eye itself often looks completely normal. However, amblyopia is the most common cause of vision loss in children, and up to three in every hundred children in the U.S. have it.[2]

This weakening will continue without early treatment, and over time, this overdependence on one eye can weaken the other to near blindness. But we can retrain our eyes to work together by addressing the eye-brain misconnection causing lazy eye and understanding how that connection extends to the whole body.

Diplopia

Double vision, or diplopia, happens when our eyes are unable to aim in the same place. As a result, they see two images of the same thing. This doubling effect can occur with images at distance or up close, and the condition is common in both children and adults.

There are two types of diplopia, monocular and binocular, and knowing which is affecting your eye is necessary in identifying the underlying cause.

. . .

If you cover one eye and the double vision goes away, but remains when you cover the other, this is likely monocular diplopia. Monocular diplopia results from damage to the eye itself, usually either the cornea or the lens.

Binocular diplopia, on the other hand, is a symptom of damage somewhere along the brain-eye connection, such as strabismus. In that cause, the two eyes are split, both in their connection to the brain and their integration with the body, creating confusion. The brain is like the traffic director that helps teach the eyes to aim together, but with two conflicting messages from the eyes, the brain has to find a way to adapt to keep directing. As a result, it normally shuts down, ignores, or suppresses the information from one eye.

Symptoms may include erratic movements of the eyes, pain in the extraorbital muscles around the eye, headaches, or nausea. Your eyes may droop from weakness, and because of the eye-body connection, you may notice body weakness that reflects the weakness in your eyes.

. . .

Diplopia can be difficult to detect, as the patient may not realize that the way he or she is seeing the world is abnormal.

An eight-year-old patient of mine was in my office recently complaining that, despite his good grades in school, he was struggling to read. In our exam, I could see his eyes as they read, skipping words and losing their place. From the outside looking in, I noticed he was having a problem tracking, but he was unaware of his erratic eye movements. As we continued talking, he asked me if it was normal to see two targets, and it all became clear. I asked how often he saw double, and he told me, "All the time."

Just like someone living with constant diplopia might never realize what it's like to see without it, many people with clear vision can't imagine what it's like to see double. This is why I made a pair of glasses that simulate double vision so others can understand the experience their loved ones are going through and be more compassionate to the ways it manifests, like difficulties at school. When the boy's father put them on, he described his brain hurting, stress levels rising, breath shortening, and chest tightening – sensations his son felt all the time when reading.

. . .

When the brain shuts off one eye to compensate for the other, you end up only using one eye to do your focusing, which makes reading, especially learning to read, very difficult. Kids may avoid reading because of their difficulty in eye coordination. If you notice your child, or even other adults, with difficulties reading and erratic eye movements, ask them, "Do you ever see double?" They may not know another option even exists until you ask.

It can be hard to track your own eye movements while reading or trying to focus, and you may not realize that seeing double isn't normal, but you may feel some other symptoms that can give you a clue that you have diplopia.

Since it can be so difficult to identify diplopia in yourself, it's a good idea to know the physical symptoms to look for in others so you can help them identify it. When you watch someone seeing double, you might notice one or both of their eyes not quite lining up. They might look crossed or slightly wandering.

In infants, eye wandering can be normal up until about three to four months old, when their eyes should look straight ahead and focus on small objects. If you still see crossing after four months, you should immediately go to a doctor because it may be a more serious condition, like a tumor. This is why the National Eye Institute recommends giving children at least one visual screening between the ages of 3 and 5 in order to detect these conditions early and address them before they can become more serious.[3]

WHAT ARE THE CAUSES?

Double vision, lazy eye, and crossed eyes are complicated conditions with potentially serious implications. Many neurological problems that could be underlying our faulty eye-brain connection go undetected long before they're discovered. In children, this can have happened during their gestation as that connection forms. The longer this eye-brain programming persists, the harder it becomes to reverse. In any case, identifying the underlying conditions that may cause these conditions is the only way to effectively treat them.

Strabismus

Crossed eyes occur most often because of a problem in a person's early physical or psychological development – whether in the uterus or after birth. The person does not know how to bring their two sides to the middle simultaneously. Crossed eyes suggest the person is turning inward, away from life because of fear, confusion, trauma, stress, or lack of developmental motor expression. The primitive survival reflexes are not integrated, and the child does not learn how to use both sides of the body with their eyes.

Early developmental problems leading to crossed eyes may be lack of movement or an irregular posture in the uterus, or birth traumas like C-section, breech position, or the use of forceps. Early infant illnesses, lack of motor exploration, or traumas of any kind may cause developmental irregularities. Even not going through the normal crawling phase can lead to confusion in the middle of the vision – and then to crossed eyes.

Other times, strabismus can develop later in life if the brain suffers some form of damage. Common causes include brain tumors, stroke, and head injuries.[4]

Amblyopia

A lazy eye results from one of the eyes being significantly weaker than the other. When this happens, the brain compensates by shutting off signals from the weaker eye and depending on the stronger one. This imbalance can result from three main causes.

- Strabismus: In cases of constant strabismus, the brain learns to tune out images from the crossed eye, and as a result, it atrophies and results in blurry vision.

- Refractive errors: If one eye has a severe refractive error, the brain will only process images from the other eye. Unlike simple refractive errors, this loss of visual acuity typically can't be treated with prescription lenses. This is because the problem is not purely a misshapen eye, but one that's complicated by an issue in the eye-brain connection.

- Cataracts or other vision loss: If one eye is out of commission due to a cataract or for another reason, the brain compensates by using only the other. If the cataract is removed, the brain may fail to process the signals that it sends.[5]

DOUBLE VISION

Diplopia can develop because of a wide variety of causes. Correctly identifying the cause of the condition is essential to determining a course of treatment.

Monocular Diplopia

Because double vision comes in two forms, let's first look at the less complicated of the two: monocular diplopia. With monocular diplopia, the double vision results from damage in the eye, either in the lens, retina, or the cornea. Since these are conditions of the eye causing diplopia, correcting them depends on healing the eye itself.

Possible causes of monocular diplopia include:

- Cataracts
- Lens dislocation
- Retinal detachment, retinal holes, or bleeding in the blood vessels of the retina
- Amblyopia
- Eye injections or surgery
- Retinal diseases like macular degeneration
- *Keratoconus,* a condition in which the abnormal thinning of the cornea causes it to become cone shaped and bulge forward in one or both eyes
- "Surfer's eye," or *pterygium,* which causes tissue growth from the conjunctiva membrane lining the eyelids and eyeball
- Corneal dystrophy
- Dry eye
- Uncorrected astigmatism
- Infections such as shingles or herpes
- Scars

Binocular Diplopia

Healing binocular diplopia is less about poor eyeball health and more about healing the eye-brain connection. The misalignment of the eyes in binocular diplopia can come from weak or underdeveloped muscles surrounding the eyes, resulting in double vision when looking in the direction of the weak muscle. However, there can also be a problem with the cranial nerves controlling them, or the connection between the nerves and the brain itself.

Underlying conditions leading to binocular diplopia include:

- **Diabetes:**
- Diabetes increases your risk of developing binocular diplopia. Diabetic eye disease can cause nerve damage that leads to double vision or eventually, potential sight loss.
- **Extraocular nerve damage:**
- Increased pressure from head trauma, infection, brain or eye tumors, a transient ischemic attack (TIA) or stroke, aneurysms, migraines, and other neurological conditions can all be causing the

extraocular nerves to misfire in their communication with the eyes.
- **Strabismus**:
- As mentioned before, having crossed eyes is a common cause of double vision. Weakened eye muscles, typically in children, result in misaligned or crossed eyes leading to double vision, and other serious medical problems if not treated
- **Myasthenia gravis:**
- This autoimmune illness can stop the nerves from directing the eye muscles, and double vision and drooping eyelids could be an early sign.
- **Graves' disease**:
- This thyroid condition can affect the eye muscles, usually resulting in vertical diplopia with one image on top of the other.
- **Multiple sclerosis (M.S.)**:
- This disease of the central nervous system can affect nerves anywhere in the brain or spinal cord, meaning it can damage the connection to the nerves that control the eyes.
- **Guillain-Barre syndrome:**
- This nerve condition causes growing weakness, first appearing in the eyes, which can manifest as double vision.
- **Sixth nerve palsy:**
- Any imbalance in the six eye muscles attached to the eyeball, the cranial nerves that innervate them

or the nerve-muscle communication can cause the nerves to stop firing, resulting in muscle weakness called a *palsy*. A palsy in the sixth cranial nerve, which controls the lateral rectus muscle on the outside of the eye, impairs the ability for the two eyes to work together, resulting in double vision, poor depth perception and even balance issues. Cranial nerve palsies can sometimes go away without treatment, but it can also create debilitating double vision. Inflammation, vascular diseases, stroke, brain tumors, infection trauma, stress and nutritional deficiencies can all play a role in causing sixth nerve palsy. If you have the symptoms, check with your doctor to rule out more serious conditions like M.S. or Parkinson's disease.

- **Stress:**
- Any systemic inflammatory response in the body, including chronic stress, will result in the swelling of the brain and a weakening of the eye-brain connection.
- **Drugs:**
- Check the side effects of any medications you may be taking. Pharmaceutical drugs and long-term antibiotics can result in anything from a mild ghost image to double vision.

WHEN SHOULD I SEE A DOCTOR?

Because of the implications these eye conditions may have on brain health, you should visit your doctor as soon as you recognize them. Not only is the condition important to diagnose to know how to treat it, but you also want to rule out any neurological problems in the brain or nerve damage. Certainly, a good eye doctor could diagnose these, but you may also want to consider visiting a neurologist to go deeper.

When you visit your eye doctor, there are a few things to bear in mind. One is that without the diagnosis of a serious condition to direct the treatment, the standard medical care for amblyopia and diplopia is, "Let's just watch it and see," which isn't a treatment at all! They may also recommend eye muscle surgery – a cosmetic cure with a cosmetic result. If the underlying problems persist, the symptoms are likely to re-emerge with time. Still, visiting a doctor is the first and most important step to diagnosing your eye condition so you can move on to the "how" in your approach to treating it.

A note about double vision: When you visit the doctor regarding double vision, it's important to be able to describe your symptoms accurately. When the eyes see double, they can see two totally separate images, but in most cases there is some level of overlap. When describing the symptoms of your type of double vision to your doctor, think about orientation, frequency, and onset. In terms of orientation, try to notice if the images appear beside one another in a horizontal plane, vertical with one hanging above the other, or oblique, a diagonal duplicate image. Diplopia can occur suddenly, affect your vision with varying degrees of severity, and last for different durations of time. Temporary double vision is less concerning and can happen from stress or fatigue. Often, the instances of diplopia are more intermittent: recurring as a symptom of an underlying condition along with other symptoms like headaches, high blood pressure, or dry eye syndrome. Of course, there can be a constant double image in your vision. This is the most concerning and likely indicative of a neurological issue or trauma.

STANDARD TREATMENTS

Once again, I recommend against treatments that address the symptoms, but not the underlying causes, of your eye condition.

One symptom-based approach a doctor may use to treat double vision is atropine eye drops, which paralyze the eye muscles. The doctor will give an eye test while a patient's focusing muscles are paralyzed and then prescribe the maximum prescription to try to force the eyes to be straight. This doesn't work and I don't recommend it! A strong prescription is a drug that makes your eyes dependent, but never heals them.

• • •

For lazy eye, the standard treatment is to patch the stronger eye to force the weaker eye to develop. But in general – I recommend against it. I have patients tell me all the time their doctor wants to patch their child for 8 hours a day, but when you patch for long periods of time, neither the child nor their brain understands the purpose of the patching. As a result, the patched eye gets lazy itself. In my clinical work, I've seen patching to be traumatic, confusing, and ineffective. When you patch a child's eye, this communicates to their brain that their midline of vision is gone. One eye can't develop better coordination with the other if it's constantly patched. Eye doctors tell children to wear patches for two to six hours a day, forcing the weaker eye to work harder, but there's no real learning in it. If you're going to use an eye patch, use it for short amounts of time or simply as a tool to exercise your eye muscles, but not enough to weaken the opposite eye.

Another option a doctor might suggest for these conditions is Botox injections, but just like surgery, these are only a temporary solution that treat the symptoms – a cosmetic cure, but not a functional one. Fixing a brain-eye problem through the eyeball doesn't work very well. This can leave behind visual difficulties with debilitating effects if the eye-brain connection is never healed. But there is no statute of limitations on brain neuroplasticity, which can heal your vision at any age.

• • •

Surgical Options

Eye muscle surgery for strabismus is the third-most common eye surgery in the US.[6] The procedure changes the eye alignment by either loosening or tightening the eye muscles. A recession surgery is when the eye muscle is detached and then reattached but further away from the front of the eye in order to weaken the muscle, while resection surgery removes a portion of the eye muscle to make it stronger.

Often doctors must go back and do multiple surgeries because the brain never gets the memo that the eye muscles were fused into place. The person remains in a state of confusion, while their brain tries to direct muscles that are now different than it remembers. This is why surgery success rates are anywhere from 30 to 80% effective. Even after surgery, the brain will still not know how to direct the muscles to aim together correctly, and confused muscle memory doesn't work so well.

THE IMPACT OF VISION THERAPY

Conventional wisdom tells us that a "critical period" exists during infancy when the brain is highly malleable, but will lose the capacity to rewire itself as it grows into adulthood. Our stereoscopic, or 3D, vision develops during this period, but most experts would say that if development is delayed beyond this critical period, the ability can never be gained. Professor Sue Barry once shared this perspective and taught it to her neurobiology students, until she underwent vision therapy and healed her own strabismus.

Dr. Barry, neurobiologist with a Ph.D. from Princeton, was born with strabismus and reversed the condition after 40 years. Surgeries at ages two, three, and seven to try and turn her eye back into place were successful in making her eyes look straight most of the time, and her vision tested at 20/20 acuity. Still, she sensed her eyes not working together. Her gaze felt jittering and unstable. When she turned 20 years old, she realized she had no stereo vision – she was only seeing in two dimensions.

She went to her eye doctor to test for it eight years later, but he told her, "You have a Ph.D. [...] You don't need stereo vision because you don't have stereo vision." She went back in her 40s, but the doctor claimed her acuity was fine, and she was likely dreaming up a problem from the traumas of her childhood surgeries. Without a solution, she started avoiding driving, making eye contact, or stretching her vision to distances where it caused the most jittering effects.

Despite three surgeries, her brain had only learned to communicate with one eye. It was negatively impacting her life, so she sought out vision therapy with optometrist Dr. Theresa Ruggiero. The input from her eyes and the receptors in her brain started exchanging correlating information and very quickly, she noticed her distance gaze stabilizing and visual clarity and sharpness improving. After six weeks, she started seeing in 3D for the first time in her life. Vision therapy had done what doctors told her was impossible – *heal her own strabismus*.[7]

As we develop, our brain has the capacity to rearrange and grow its neural networks to accommodate new information, like learning a new skill or reacting to environmental or interpersonal stressors. This behavior is called neuroplasticity, and since the eyes originate from brain tissue, they have the same capacity for regrowth as the brain, even late into life, as Dr. Barry's example demonstrates.

This is why my number one recommendation, and the only treatment that actually works, for correcting the muscle imbalances that lead to double vision, crossed eyes, and lazy eye is vision therapy. The two eyes aren't working together, and the brain is confused. That eye-brain connection is what needs to be restored. Vision therapy encourages the brain to use its plasticity to relearn how to use both eyes together without strong prescriptions, injections, or surgeries.

Through the eye-brain re-education process of vision therapy, both eyes and the brain all learn to start aiming together. These practices help improve visual coordination skills and plasticity of the eyes through their cooperation with the brain. In my 35 years treating strabismus with vision therapy, I've seen how much more lasting and effective of a treatment it is than surgery. It changes people's lives.

If your eye doctor tells you that there's not much they can do about your condition, seek out a holistic eye doctor who might be more knowledgeable in alternative treatments, or at least give you a second opinion about your options.

See the end of this chapter for my full eye exercise protocol for these conditions.

OTHER TREATMENT OPTIONS

While vision therapy is my number one recommendation for training the eyes to work together, there are other treatments that can improve your condition.

· · ·

Acupuncture

Acupuncture has been shown to serve as a useful complement in treating amblyopia,[8] and one 2010 study found acupuncture to have the same, if not superior, treatment effect for amblyopia in children as patching.[9] A 2014 case study determined acupuncture likely to be a helpful treatment for diplopia that occurs with sixth nerve palsy.[10]

Craniosacral therapy

In my practice, I encourage patients with these eye muscle imbalances to seek out craniosacral therapy, which can be very effective in releasing tension patterns or trauma in the eyes, brain, and body. It can also help improve your strabismus and lazy eye. Research has suggested the practice is the perfect complement for the elderly, children, and other fragile populations to release fascial restrictions and improve muscular outcomes.[11]

Therapeutic Prism (TP) Prescriptions

Therapeutic prism lenses are often used to address binocular double vision problems. The only kind of prisms you should use are called "yoked" prisms, which shift your spatial awareness and expand your peripheral vision. (Other lenses may attempt to fix your eyes by forcing them into one position, which you should avoid.)

Yoked prisms improve depth perception, eye tracking, eye-brain communication, and sports performance. You may even notice results in your posture, balance, coordination, and cognition in the process. Some eye doctors prescribe them for daily wear, but this way they become a crutch. Instead, I recommend them as a tool to use in combination with your vision therapy.

Color Therapy

Anything that narrows our visual field, and our peripheral vision will result in more double vision, but color therapy helps open up the whole retina, which can have the opposite effect. Find a holistic doctor who knows about color therapy and can prescribe the proper colors to re-sensitize the retinal cells in your eyes that have been shut down. As your peripheral vision opens, you'll have more vision to engage your eyes, leading to a quick reduction in your double vision. (See Chapter 9 for more information about color therapy.)

Diet

As always, ensuring proper eye nutrition will help boost its systemic and metabolic processes, resulting in greater eye-brain cooperation. Make sure to get enough eye-healthy trace minerals like magnesium, chromium, and selenium, and antioxidants like beta-carotene and lutein. Several studies have shown lutein's capacity to preserve neural efficiency and improve cognitive performance,[12] which can be helpful in restoring the eye-brain connection. In animal studies, bilberries have been shown to inhibit stress-related gene expressions in the retina,[13] and supplementation of bilberry extract may prevent eye fatigue.[14]

Taurine is the most abundant amino acid in the retina. It plays a role in cell hydration, digestion, mineral regulation, immune health, and antioxidant function, as well as central nervous system and eye function. Studies show it may protect against the degeneration of retinal ganglion cells.[15] Deficiency can lead to visual dysfunction and retinal lesions.[16]

When the goal is to restore muscle balance through eye and brain health, consume vitamins and minerals that support brain, muscle, and eye health, particularly omega-3 fatty acids and zinc.

EYE EXERCISES FOR EYE COORDINATION

The vision therapy I administer in my practice includes visual tracking, focusing, and coordination exercises. Eye patching as a tool to restore vision, eye dialogue to uncover hidden misperceptions in your eyes, and the animal eye chart exercise will all help to disrupt the conflicting pattern between the eyes.

Of course, it takes regular practice, and won't happen overnight. According to "Stereo Sue" Barry who restored her own stereo vision, "The more I practiced, the more I progressed. [...] Doing just a little bit each day was very powerful. So I didn't have to change my life to do vision therapy, but I did have to put aside a small part of my life to do the therapy on a regular basis and I pretty much did it every day."[17]

A little bit goes a long way, so start with what you can, but know the more you incorporate into your daily life, the more impactful your progress will be. When you're ready, below is my 90-day protocol for helping eyes coordinate with one another. Each day, exercises should be done twice – once in the morning and once in the evening. This exercise protocol is preventative in nature, so repeat again in another 90 days for continued eye resilience.

(Find the full description of these exercises on my website: https://www.drsamberne.com/eye-exercises/)

VITAL VISION

DAYS 1-7

- Figure 8 Eye Massage
- N Breath and Palm Hum
- Sunning

DAYS 8-14

- Eye Dialogue
- Tongue Clock Palming

DAY 15-21

- Moro Reflex Integration
- Tonic Labyrinth Reflex Integration
- Eye Brain Body Fun

DAYS 22-30

- Figure 8 Eye Massage
- The Thumb Game

171

DAYS 31-37

- Sunning
- N Breath and Palm Hum

DAYS 38-46

- Yin Yang Chart
- Tongue Clock

DAYS 47-53

- Sunning
- Eye Dialogue
- Eye Brain Body Fun

DAYS 54-60

- Moro Reflex Integration
- The Thumb Game
- N Breath and Palm Hum

DAYS 61-69

- Tonic Labyrinth Reflex Integration
- Sunning
- Eye Brain Body Fun

DAYS 70-76

- Eye Dialogue
- The Thumb Game
- Figure 8 Eye Massage

DAYS 77-81

- Long Swings
- Moro Reflex Integration
- Yin Yang Chart

DAYS 82-90

- N Breath and Palm Hum
- Eye Brain Body Fun
- Figure 8 Eye Massage

CHAPTER 7
DRUGS AND SURGERY VERSUS HERBS AND AROMATHERAPY

One recurring theme in this book is that prescription drugs and surgeries may seem to eliminate eye conditions – but they come with side effects and leave the underlying causes untouched. Fortunately, you can tap into the body's own healing powers and assist them using plant-based essential oils without the risks associated with drugs.

WHAT IS THE OCULAR MICROBIOME?

One area of eye health that can neglected or harmed by common pharmaceutical treatments is the ocular microbiome. Microbiota – that is, bacteria, fungi, and viruses – outnumber our own cells in our body by 10 to one! These naturally occurring microbes live together in communities called microbiomes, and they are critical in staving off diseases. Keeping the right balance of microbes in these microbiome communities helps our immune system and enables proper digestion and metabolism. On the other hand, reductions in microbiome diversity are associated with several diseases.[1] The gut, skin, and oral and nasal cavities all have their own unique microbiome communities that form early in life, but change depending on factors like diet, medications, and environmental exposure.

In 1930, Dr. Robert Keilty was the first to describe the eye's microbiome when he discovered a small subset of ocular bacteria from a culture analysis of tissue swabs off the surface of the eye and interior eyelids.[2] Researchers continued to dig into Keiltey's findings and in 1975, they positively identified bacteria strains, mainly *Staphylococcus* and *Propionibacterium*, in 90% of eye samples. A 2016 culture analysis found the eye microbiome to also contain viruses and fungi.[3]

Recent evidence indicates that the collection of ocular microbiota protects the eyes from infections, while any imbalance can increase the risk of developing ocular diseases.[4] [5] A 2002 study suggested that the eye's microbiota have a role in mucin metabolism, an enzyme that aids in waste removal.[6] This is an important link considering the role of waste accumulation in most eye conditions, especially AMD. A 2007 study compared healthy eyes with those diagnosed with dry eye syndrome and found 97% of dry eye patients had positive bacterial cultures, as opposed to only 75% of healthy eyes.[7]

The ocular microbiome includes microbes in the cornea and the clear conjunctival epithelium covering the eye. This serves as both a barrier to ocular infection and a point of interface between skin microbiota, including from the lashes and eyelids, and the surface of the eye. This communication is critical for ocular homeostasis and immune functioning.

The ocular biome is directly connected to the gut. The gut-retina axis is a network of nerves that connects the enteric nervous system of the gut with the nerves of the eyes. Recent studies have indicated that a disruption to gut microbiota sends inflammatory signals to the eyes along this axis.[8] Uveitis, inflammation in the middle layer of the eye wall, is linked to gastrointestinal disorders like ulcerative colitis and Crohn's disease.[9] A 2017 study found that the body's microbiome can cause the gut to signal retina-specific T cells, the most important white blood cells in our immune systems, to trigger inflammation in the eyes of mice.[10]

As you can see, keeping the eye's microbiome in balance is important for eye health, but many treatments negatively impact it. Contact lenses can alter the delicate status of the ocular microbiome. A 2002 study found that colony forming units (CFUs) and bacterial species diversity increase when wearing contacts.[11] In 2016, researchers found contact lenses may alter the conjunctive microbial structure, accounting for an increased risk for eye conditions such as giant papillary conjunctivitis and keratitis.[12]

As we continue to investigate the physiological interactions of these ecosystems, our understanding of the ocular microbiome will likely follow the same parallel as the gut. Throughout the 20th century, we knew pathogenic microbes could cause gut dysfunction, but the focus was identifying and prescribing antibiotics to kill them. Now, our awareness has shifted to nourishing a healthy microbiome ecosystem as preventative medicine. In the same way, as our awareness continues to shift towards a holistic view of the body, we'll increasingly discover that protecting the delicate balance of our ocular microbiomes can prevent and even reverse ocular diseases.

Antibiotic Resistance

Yet despite our growing understanding of the body's need for microbiomes, antibiotic use is on the rise. At the same time, the discovery of new antibiotics has slowed, leading to more strains of antibiotic-resistant bacteria that researchers are unable to cure. The CDC calls antibiotic resistance "one of the greatest public health challenges of our time, [causing] illnesses that were once easily treatable [...] to become dangerous infections."[13] A 2014 report cited antimicrobial resistance (AMR) claims at least 50,000 lives per year in Europe and the U.S. alone, a number that experts estimate will be closer to 10 million by 2050.[14]

One area where the concern over antibiotic resistance is affecting is in another traditional option for restoring health: surgical procedures. According to Dr. Harvey Fishman, most intraocular surgeries result in infections because foreign bacteria get introduced into the ocular system through either the lashes, the eyelid margin, or in the cornea.[15] Doctors traditionally administer preoperative antibiotics before surgery to reduce the risk of postoperative infections, but little is known about the role of these antibiotics on the bodily microbiomes. Considering how much they impact our gut microbiota, it's safe to say antibiotics likely alter our ocular microbiota, and the jarring effects of surgery likely expound those effects. For example, cataract surgery has been shown to have a significant effect on the bacterial composition of the ocular microbiome for weeks after the procedure, even after completing an antibiotic regimen.[16] This is yet another reason to avoid eye surgery if at all possible!

THE BODY HEALS

The business of pharmaceutical drugs and surgical treatments benefits from simply covering up the cause of illness, but medical experts with a genuine desire to heal have taken a renewed interest in the powers of ancient medicinal essences. Increasingly, research is showing us that we don't need to kill, drug, or cut our natural anatomy to heal it. In fact, under the right conditions, we're learning that the body can heal itself.

One exciting topic in the world of eye health is ocular regeneration. Scientists have known for years that the brain forms new neuronal cells, a process called *neurogenesis*, and now, evidence is indicating that retinal nerve cells are potentially able to regenerate, re-vitalize, and replenish themselves. A 2017 National Eye Institute study found that neurogenesis also occurs in the retinal ganglion cells (RGCs), which are responsible for transmitting information from the eyes to the brain.[17] A 2017 animal study found that cells within an injured mouse's eye can be induced into regenerating neurons that integrate themselves into the eye's circuitry.[18] And in 2018, depleted immune cells in mice retinas reproduced themselves and returned to their original arrangement and functions.[19]

. . .

In one study, boosting brain-derived neurotrophic factor (BDNF) levels in the eye after optic nerve injury significantly improved RGC survival and function in cats.[20] BDNF is a protein that plays a role in stimulating the growth of neurons in the central nervous system, and in studies, patients with higher levels of BDNF had a lower risk of developing neurodegenerative disorders like Alzheimer's and dementia.[21] Research has found that natural remedies, like curcumin, the bioactive compound found in turmeric, is effective in boosting BDNF levels,[22] and adding more trace minerals like zinc to your diet may modulate BDNF activity.[23]

One way to boost eye cell regeneration could be through prebiotic fiber. Gut bacteria convert prebiotics into butyrate, which a 2019 animal study showed to increase BDNF.[24] Research into probiotic eye drops has only just begun, but in one study, a four-week treatment resulted in modest improvements in symptoms of vernal keratoconjunctivitis, a chronic allergy inflammatory disease affecting the ocular surface, with no side effects.[25]

ESSENTIAL OILS

Another promising area of research is the use of essential oils and herbs for eye health. While the power of these treatments may need more research to confirm, my experience as an eye care practitioner supports the science that already exists. Countless patients have reversed, slowed down, and healed their eye conditions with a natural, holistic approach instead of drugs or surgery. It's my firm belief that the more medical investigators continue to explore essential oils as a complementary medicine, the more likely they are to uncover their full potential as the future of medicine. Since the health of the eyes is connected to the health of other bodily systems, essential oils can be an invaluable addition to holistic eye care.

Essential oils are concentrated plant extracts machine-pressed or distilled that can come from flower, leaves, bark, roots, berries, seeds and/or fruit. They retain the smell, flavor, unique chemical composition, and vital nutrient profiles as the source plant, but in concentrated quantities. Their medicinal properties vary from plant to plant.

Their rich and complex blend of naturally occurring minerals, vitamins, antioxidants, and other nutrients allows essences to help restore our systemic balance, setting limits on the behavior of a disease or disorder. Essential oils are also adaptogenic, meaning they have the flexibility to respond to our individual needs and adapt to the ever-changing organisms that affect our health. Plant essences are antibacterial and antioxidant, support the immune system, and provide oxygenation and hydration to cells. Some have even antiviral and antifungal properties.

You may not think of yourself as someone who would use essential oils as medicine, but if you ever rubbed a cough suppressant on your chest, then eucalyptus, cedar leaf, and nutmeg oils were likely among the active ingredients in your relief.

Aromatic oils have been a part of human medicine for thousands of years, treating ailments like bronchitis, pneumonia, pharyngitis, diarrhea, periodontal disease, and wounds. Oils were widely used in ancient Egypt as a treatment for infection, and the ancient Hebrews referred to myrrh as "holy oil," more valuable than gold.

Many are familiar with the story of the wise men who brought frankincense and myrrh to Jesus after his birth. But these oils are more than just perfumes. They've been used treat wounds, inflammation, cystitis, rheumatic joints, skin sores, bleeding, fungal infections, burns, pharyngitis, syphilis, and leprosy.[26] Studies have shown that these two oils are even more powerful when combined together.[27] The wise men were wise indeed to bring such powerful oils as gifts!

Yet, while they've been a part of medicinal practice for centuries, there are many difficulties in researching the effectiveness of aromatherapy and plant essences. If oils yield improvements, it can be hard to separate the effectiveness of the oil from other environmental triggers, the massage or therapeutic method of application, or even an olfactory memory from childhood changing mental behaviors. Aromatic substances in blind studies present problems to the scientific process and essence variations from plant to plant, region to region and even through extraction and storage methods. In other words, there are too many variables for the scientific community to be convinced.

Furthermore, studies about the efficacy of pharmaceutical drugs are usually well-funded by the pharmaceutical companies that produces the drugs. These companies make more money off synthetic products than they would natural products that are difficult to patent. As a result, funds are not devoted to studying the efficacy of essential oils.

What the Science Says

Even without major funding into the medical uses of plant essences, we have a strong collection of research that indicates the powerful medicinal potential of essential oils. Let's take a closer look at what the science says about several key effects of essential oils and their impact on eye health.

Anti-Diabetic

Keeping diabetes under control reduces the risk of nearly all major eye conditions. In animal studies, rosemary (*Rosmarinus officinalis*) demonstrated hyperglycemic and insulin release inhibitory effects,[28] and low concentrations of lemon balm oil served as an efficient hypoglycemic agent.[29]

Anti-inflammatory, Antioxidant

Inflammation is another risk factor for eye conditions, particularly AMD. A 2003 study confirmed that the traditional use of lavender in Iranian folk medicine is effective at treating inflammatory diseases and pain.[30] In animal studies, the antioxidant effects of peppermint oil were shown to protect the kidneys and liver against carbon tetrachloride, one of the main environmental toxins associated with cellular liver damage.[31] An examination of 50 essential oils in 2011 found that all increased bodily nitric oxide production, which is produced by nearly every cell and critical for blood vessel health.

Antimicrobial

Several essential oils can boost the body's response to bacteria, viruses, and fungi – all of which have the potential to impact eye health. Particularly when it comes to eye surgery, reducing the risk of infection is essential.

A topical treatment of eucalyptus, tea tree, thyme, clove, and some citrus species has demonstrated antimicrobial effects against infection following surgery, and researchers see it as a simple and inexpensive potential alternative to long-term systemic antibiotic therapy.[32]

Peppermint[33] and sandalwood oils[34] have shown strong antiviral activity against the Herpes simplex viruses-1 and -2. Tea tree oil was shown to significantly inhibit the replicative cycle in the early stages of the influenza virus.[35] Studies have found strong bactericidal activity in tea tree oil,[36] and oregano, and thyme oils.[37] The antifungal activity of tea tree oil[38] and thyme oil[39] have been shown to be an effective treatment against strains of candida.

Digestion

As gut health is directly tied to the ocular microbiome, good digestion helps to keep eyes healthy. After four weeks of a peppermint oil treatment, patients with irritable bowel syndrome (IBS) reported improved abdominal symptoms.[40] Aromatherapy with peppermint oil effectively reduced perceived nausea following surgery.[41] Fennel seed oil has been shown to reduce intestinal spasms and increase motility of the small intestine in infants with colic.[42]

Beyond the Science

As promising as the science behind essential oils is, their impact on our wellbeing goes even deeper. Countless times, my clients express how much more improvement they see in their healing process when their efforts are applied in conjunction with essential oils. They're always amazed to see their symptoms diminish and to feel more self-connected. This is because, in addition to their ability to heal physically, medicinal essences can help awaken our connection to Mother Earth and the spiritual.

Medicinal essences are to the tree or plant as blood is to our human bodies. Just like blood, plant essences are concentrated with vitamins and minerals that circulate through the plant body, and they carry their own temperature, aroma, and taste. Just as the blood carries life that can be transfused to save a dying body, plant essences carry natural healing powers that give life when consumed. In harnessing the natural power of plant essences, we connect more deeply to our own healing powers. This is why the more deeply we connect to nature and our bodies, the more effectively the essences will work.

Depending on the plant part from which the essence was extracted, each essence will affect the body in different ways. Rose, for example, comes from the flower, which brings your heart chakra into balance for giving and receiving love and joy and a sense of inner peace. Seeds, like sweet fennel, are for new beginnings. Essences from tree bark are good for resolving boundary issues, and root essences can make you feel more grounded.

As we'll discuss more in Chapter 9, all living things are surrounded by an energy field that contains patterns of information, which tools like a gas discharge visualization (GDV) camera can detect, and essential oils have the highest measured energy frequency of any natural substance. Whereas the energy fields of a body with normal, healthy energy systems, read at about 63 mHz, rose vibrates at over 300 mHz, helichrysum at 120 mHz, cypress at 118 mHz, juniper berry at 117 mHz, and frankincense at 115 mHz. Higher frequency energies are able to destroy lower frequency energies, which is why essential oils are so effective against pathogens in the human body. Their energetic vibrations introduce the healing power of light to the body, mind, and spirit.

. . .

When you measure the energy discharge of essential oils, their vibration and photon emissions are also more uniform and brighter than those measured from pharmaceuticals, which have a much lower frequency. Scientists measured essential oils with an oscilloscope to find they significantly raised energy levels above average, and biophysicists have found essential oils to protect, repair, and clean the human energy field.

HOW TO CHOOSE AN ESSENTIAL OIL

DISCLAIMER:

If you have questions or are concerned for any reason – if the person being treated is larger or smaller than average, in poor health, pregnant, or very young or old – it is best to work with an experienced medicinal aromatherapist until you have developed depth in this area. For more information about using medicinal essential oils, see my book I Sense: At Play in the Field of Healing.

There are many essential oil companies cropping up across the country, but some will produce better results than others. The first key to picking an essential oil is finding a reputable aromatherapy company. Find small family farms that use essences as medicines for themselves so you can trust that they understand the complexities of extracting, handling, and storing them. Look for one that practices wild crafting or biodynamic farming, which involve less manual and mechanical interventions in care and harvesting and add great value to the power and resonance of an essence.

Not every essential oil has the vibrational levels and chemical complexities right from the plant that a therapeutic quality oil needs to effectively stimulate healing. In other words, the form in which you take the oil matters. Bath salts and candles may claim to have a touch of certain essential oils, but they won't help therapeutically. The more an essential essence is treated or chemically adulterated, the lower its profound healing effect, so avoid pre-mixed blends or essences stored in carrier oils.

How to Apply an Essential Oil

Once you've chosen your essential oil, using it correctly will help you derive the most benefit. Before you apply, first I recommend what I call a "meet-and-greet" experience. Open the oil and just breathe it in. Start slowly. The goal is to connect to the rhythms of the vital plant energies and nourish your depleted self. Breathe in a deep inhale through your nose of the aroma and ask yourself how it hits you. Take time to analyze how you feel and what you experience. Your olfactory sense connects very deeply to the limbic system, the emotional brain, so if you feel a positive response of "Yes, I can do this," at the scent, then you're ready to go.

In my experience, the most powerful and effective way of absorbing the essence's energy is topically, directly on the skin and without a carrier oil, undiluted. Applied directly to the body, essential oils offer a high degree of oxygenation, hydration, and detoxification. It is possible that some essences may cause skin irritation as a reaction to the essence itself or as a detoxification reaction, so always start with a test patch when using a new essence. Put a drop or two on your forearm and monitor the reaction for a couple of minutes. Skin tissue is a major dumping ground for hidden toxicities, so most people will experience some reaction the essences, such as itchiness, irritation, or rashes, especially as a detoxification. If you have a reaction, see if there is an essence to neutralize it and try a reduced dosage that the skin can handle without irritation.

If you at any time you experience more burning than makes you feel comfortable, don't try to wash it away with water. Instead, get a carrier oil and apply it right on the area that burns, and you'll feel relief. My top recommendations are argan, jojoba, or prickly pear oil.

Once you've done your test patch, take a drop of your first oil and place it at the hairline on either side, another drop on each temple, and one on each cheek. Massage each drop gently into the skin. Then, close your eyes and again, take a breath or two to notice how you feel. Go deeper, further inside and uncover what you feel. Movement, temperature, activation, circulation – whatever words best describe the sensations you experience, give them a name, and identify them.

To apply more than one essential oil, I find the most effective application method to be a layering technique. Massage the second essence right on top of the previous one so they work synergistically, and again, close your eyes, and smell and experience the oil. Then, layer on another and repeat the process. With each layer, apply slightly less to keep the area you cover within the boundaries of the essence underneath. Layering is the best way to get the synergistic benefits of multiple oils while taking advantage of the unique vibrational energy and healing power of each essence, which can be negatively disrupted when pre-mixed.

Some essences have a *yin*, or cool quality, while others are *yang*, or hot, like oregano or clove bud, and can be more irritating. Follow a "cold-hot-cold" pattern to safely apply oils of different temperature qualities anywhere on the body. I recommend always beginning and ending with a yin (cool) quality oil, with hot oils in between.

When using aromatherapy for treating any condition, the rule is to apply the essences directly onto the area of concern or as close to it as possible, but keep away from the mouth, eyes, and mucous membranes. For digestive issues, for example, I would recommend four drops on the stomach area over the digestive tract, twice a day for about two weeks. For eye conditions, however, you should never put the oils directly into your eyes. Instead, apply the oils around the outside of each socket a safe distance away. If a drop gets into your eyes, don't worry. It may be an uncomfortable 15 to 30 minutes, but they won't cause any damage. You can attempt to neutralize the discomfort with a carrier oil, but only apply it around the eye socket, never directly in the eye. You can also use eye compresses like chamomile and fennel, which are great for reducing inflammation.

MY ESSENTIAL OILS EYE PROTOCOL

In my years of study, practice, and experience, I have established an optimal essential oil protocol for eye health. Each oil should be applied in the indicated order for maximum effect. Follow this daily practice in conjunction with your eye exercises, diet, and lifestyle changes for significant improvement in your healing journey.

. . .

Follow this protocol once a day in the beginning and see how you do with it. You'll likely find your vision to be brighter, with particular improvements in night vision. If you have an eye condition and are following other diet, exercise, and lifestyle protocols to address it, you'll quickly start to notice relief in your symptoms. If you sense some peripheral vision expansion, try to move the practice to twice a day.

#1. Fennel:

This herb has been used for centuries by some of the most ancient civilizations, including Rome, Greece, India, and Egypt. Fennel benefits digestive and stomach health, but it also invigorates the kidney and spleen and helps with self-expression. You may recognize this hardy plant for its licorice flavor or feathery leaves, but the essential oil is extracted from the seeds, which is why fennel is the first in this protocol. Known for new beginnings, birthing and the start of something new, fennel seed oil opens us up to opportunities and brings the energy of new birth, death, and rebirth. Apply around your face and eyes to open your sight and reduce tunnel vision. This oil is *yin*, or cool, but when you apply it, you'll likely feel a little warmth.

. . .

#2. Carrot seed:

Just like carrots, this essential oil is great for the skin. This second essence is also from a seed, again indicating change, newness, beginnings, and birth. Carrot seed oil is also a blood purifier and supports gallbladder health. All of these functions together help to hydrate and oxygenate the eye tissue. When you apply this second oil after the fennel, you'll notice a slightly warmer sensation.

#3 Frankincense:

Extracted from the resin of a small tree, frankincense not only supports a balanced nervous system, it's a major visual opener. When you apply this oil after the carrot seed oil, you will feel it stimulating stagnant energy with an uplifting and freeing sensation. As a relief from the warmth of the first two oils, frankincense is a little cooler.

#4. Laurel leaf:

In Greece, laurel leaves adorn the holy temples and circular wreaths of the plant were used to crown victors in the ancient Olympic games. This is why I call laurel leaf the "Queen of the lymph system," because of its ability to support lymphatic health. This oil extract comes from the leaves and branches of an evergreen shrub and has uplifting qualities that spark our inner vision. In addition to using laurel leaf after frankincense in this eye protocol, I recommend a drop or two on the heart before you take a shower for an instant spirit uplifting, as the water will push the oil deeper into your body.

#5. Hydrosol Helichrysum:

I recommend hydrosol helichrysum rather than a pure helichrysum essential oil because the pure oil is extremely expensive. The hydrosol is a less concentrated version that retains the frequency of the essential oil for a fraction of the cost. It's high vibrational, anti-inflammatory, great for the skin, and uplifting to the heart. It reduces inflammation on the eyelids and hydrates the eye to improve symptoms of dry eye computer vision syndrome.

CHAPTER 8
NUTRITION TIPS – WHAT TO EAT FOR HEALTHY EYES

Whenever there's a problem in the eye, nine times out of ten, the cause can be found somewhere in the patient's diet. The foods of today are becoming increasingly over-processed and void of significant nutritional quality. Big food corporations sell products laced with simple sugars and artificial ingredients promoted as "healthy," while pushing food behaviors that simultaneously promote fatphobia and obesity. As a result, we consume too many carbs and have generally poor dietary absorption.

A person can eat the most wholesome diet in the world, but if their body is unable to produce a full range of dietary enzymes, it never fully absorbs those nutrients. Malabsorption can be caused by an inflammatory diet, poor gut health, or other conditions – so ensuring the health of all body systems will boost nutritional status.

The eye conditions macular degeneration, glaucoma, cataracts, and dry eye syndrome are all usually symptoms of bigger problems that are manifesting in the eyes. To address these symptoms, we need to find the underlying systemic problem that is cutting your eyes off from sufficient oxygenation and hydration and allowing for the build-up of waste. If the foods that you eat are adding to these systemic problems, they're also accelerating the damage in your eyes.

What we eat, our brain, and our vision are all connected. This chapter will highlight some of the ways you can boost your eye-brain function through nutrition, as well as the upkeep of a healthy "second brain," the gastrointestinal tract. At the end is a glossary of nutrients for improved eye, brain, and gut health that you can reference as needed in each step along your journey to healing your vision.

THE STATE OF DIETS TODAY

Until you make a conscious effort to eat well, you're probably missing out on some serious nutrition. The typical Western diet – categorized by a higher intake of red and processed meats, high-fat dairy, eggs, fried foods, and refined grains – is associated with a markedly higher risk of AMD and other eye conditions.[1] This high-fat diet causes inflammatory gut microbiota to induce hyperglycemia, which damages the retinal blood vessels and cuts off circulation.

Most of us are unable to properly metabolize carbs because of mineral imbalances and blood sugar levels, and we don't even know it. As a result, sugar molecules often remain in our blood, increasing the risk of candida, arthritis, obesity, pre-diabetic conditions, and diabetes, as well as major cellular and energetic problems. Artificial sweeteners trick the body into starvation mode, holding onto calories from other foods and converting them to more fat. That is why diet soda is just as likely to result in obesity as its full-sugar counterpart.[2]

High fructose corn syrup (HFCS) is made from the overproduced and highly subsidized genetically modified corn that has made its way into virtually every processed food item today. This sweetener contains water, glucose, and higher quantities of fructose than table sugar. In the early 2000s, 25% of the average American's calorie consumption came from sugars, mostly fructose.[3] In 2009, people in the U.S. were averaging 50 grams of HFCS a day, and one study found that, per gram, they were likely consuming up to 0.57 micrograms of the toxic metal mercury along with it.[4] A 2010 study by the American Association for Cancer Research found fructose to better facilitate the proliferation of cancer cells than glucose, while avoiding HFCS may disrupt cancer cell growth.[5]

Our gastrointestinal tract is unable to properly absorb HFCS, but the pancreas and liver still ramp up for metabolism. This can cause unhealthy fat production in the liver. This can lead to non-alcoholic fatty liver disease, a condition virtually unknown before 1980, but now affecting up to 30% of American adults as consumption levels of HFCS rise. Not only can HFCS consumption lead to cirrhosis of the liver, but it also promotes the build-up of visceral fat around the organs, increases blood pressure, LDL ("bad" cholesterol), and the production of cancer-causing free radicals. Several studies have linked non-alcoholic fatty liver disease to cardiovascular disease, hypertension, and diabetes.[6]

Most people have at least some sensitivity to gluten without even knowing it, so cutting it out will likely improve your health. A diet high in gluten can lead to poor thyroid function, a slower metabolism, decreased immune function and poor detoxification systems, increasing the body's inflammatory response, and contributing to autoimmune conditions. ADHD, anxiety, autism, autoimmune disorders, brain fog, digestive disorders, seizures, sugar cravings, and skin breakouts of all kinds can be signs of an unaddressed gluten intolerance. Instead of wheat, couscous, bulgur, semolina, spelt, rye, kamut, or barley, which all contain gluten, try alternatives like amaranth, arrowroot, buckwheat, corn, millet, quinoa, and rice.

Our diets have also become increasingly acidic, which can create excess acidity in the body that allows for the growth of disease. Chronic inflammation, weight gain and obesity, diabetes, kidney conditions, weakened immunity, premature aging, osteoporosis, weak or brittle bones, fractures, and endocrine imbalances can all result from too much acid. Consuming less protein, processed foods, flours, sugar, coffee, tea, and alcohol can decrease your systemic acidity. Every morning, drink a half a lemon in water – once digested and metabolized, lemon juice produces alkaline byproducts, which make the urine more alkaline. Incorporate more dark leafy greens like kale, spinach, collards or bok choy into your meals. Miso or veggie broth are also great pH balancers.

Inflammation is at the root of many of today's health problems, and an overly acidic environment keeps the inflammation going indefinitely. The immune system causes inflammation as a protective response to harmful stimuli, but as a long-term response it leads to disease and deterioration. Cellular inflammation causes swelling, pain, and toxicity, which may manifest as symptoms like infection, joint pain, digestive disorders, anxiety, headaches, depression, and allergies. Inflammation in the brain is what leads to degenerative diseases like Alzheimer's or Parkinson's, and long-term inflammation inhibits the body's ability to process metabolic waste, causing an accumulation in the cells and increasing oxidative stress.

An unhealthy diet is more than just junk food, it's also the toxic products we consume:

- Processed meats and cold cuts are class 1 carcinogens.
- Canola oil is highly processed at a high heat with deodorants that cover up how often it goes rancid, which when consumed, can be toxic.
- Many U.S.-produced cheeses contain aluminum as an additive, which is everywhere in our cookware, food packaging, and deodorants, but toxic to the nervous system.
- Peanut butter may contain the mold aflatoxin B1, a classified Group 1 carcinogen that targets the liver and can lead to cancer.[7] Instead, choose almond butter for a safer and healthier option.

GUT HEALTH AND VISION

Think of the gastrointestinal system as the body's second nervous system: its second brain. According to professor

Dr. Micheal Gershon, author of the book, *The Second Brain*, "The bowel has got to work right, or no one will have the luxury to think at all."[8] We already know the eyes have their own microbiome, but they also have a lymphatic system, emphasizing this intimate connection they have with the gut.

Toxins, antibiotics, herbicides, and pesticides have caused many of us to lose our network of good gut bacteria that protect it from inflammation. Your body can react to bad food with a quick inflammatory reaction intended to control the damage, but when that inflammation is constant, it compromises intestinal permeability and leads to a condition called "leaky gut." A diet high in processed foods, salt, sugars, unhealthy fats, and artificial ingredients can add to this chronic inflammatory response. Since that diet is also low in nutrients, the cells have no energy to remove toxins, making the body even more susceptible to illness.

Our gut health affects our emotional health and overall perceptions – which, as we've seen, are tied to our visual abilities. The vagus nerve provides a direct line of two-way communication, which is why improving gastrointestinal health has a positive influence on behavior. With over 90% of the mood regulator serotonin produced in the gut and a hundred million nerve cells lining the GI tract, it should come as no surprise that stress and anxiety in the mind can affect the gut, and vice versa. The gut also produces dopamine, norepinephrine, acetylcholine, and gamma-Aminobutyric acid (GABA), which play critical roles in controlling mood, concentration, learning, and drive.

On the other hand, studies have shown how low-inflammatory diets, like the Mediterranean diet, can reduce the symptoms of depression,[9] and researchers classified 12 antidepressant nutrients in certain foods, like spinach, romaine lettuce, cauliflower, and strawberries.[10] Studies have shown that introducing beneficial gut flora by taking probiotics can mitigate anxiety and symptoms of depression with equal effectiveness of prescription medications, but without the side effects of disrupting the gut balance.[11]

The gut contains 70% of the immune system, so greater efforts to improve your gut health will result in more marked improvements in overall health. I recommend adding one or more strains of prebiotic fiber to your diet, like *Bifidobacterium* and *Lactobacillus plantarum*. These strains prevent the adhesion of bad bacteria and help to produce short-chain fatty acids to nourish the intestinal cells. Carbon redox molecules are a natural product of healthy internal flora that maintain the intestinal lining, increasing gut health and reducing inflammation, and you can take supplements as a good way to improve dietary absorption.

Eat plain, unpasteurized yogurt without sugar, or other fermented foods like sauerkraut, kim chi or natto. Eat the superfoods above for high levels of antioxidants, which may improve the gut microbiota,[12] or Jerusalem artichokes, cocoa, jicama, almonds, Brazil nuts, raspberries, pumpkin, and taro to maintain your gut health. A diet high in the antioxidant vitamins C and E, as well as selenium and retinoic acid, can mitigate mucosal inflammation and transform the gut microbiota towards an anti-inflammatory profile.[13]

Synthetic additives, colorants, and flavorings, HFCS and other artificial sweeteners, oxidized and GMO vegetable oils, grain-fed meats, gluten and hybridized wheat, crops with glyphosate pesticides, and processed dairy all disrupt the gut microbiome, and should be avoided as much as possible.

DIET, VISION, AND NUTRIENT ABSORPTION

Compared to the rest of the body, the eyes have very high metabolic needs. To carry out their necessary cellular processes, the vascular tissue of the eye demands sufficient nutrients. But the delicate distribution system of microcapillaries makes it vulnerable to damage under conditions of even minor change. This is why how we eat affects how we see – the entire process of digestion, absorption, and elimination of what we eat has an impact on our vision.

Normally, eating triggers the release of digestive enzymes in the stomach and intestinal tract that break the food down into simpler forms so it can be absorbed into the bloodstream. The blood distributes the nutrients throughout the body as needed, and whatever remains in excess is expelled during your next trip to the bathroom. *Malabsorption syndrome* occurs when any part of that process is interrupted: the enzymes needed to break down food are inhibited in their function or production, or your lymphatic system fails to carry and distribute nutrients appropriately.

Some specific conditions of the intestine, liver, or pancreas, like celiac disease or chronic pancreatitis, can cause malabsorption. Severe congestive heart failure can result in a bowel wall too swollen with fluid to absorb nutrients well. With cystic fibrosis, the body produces a thick mucus that disrupts not only lung health, but digestive health as well, which can result in malabsorption syndrome. Bacteria, viruses or parasites can cause direct damage to the intestinal wall and lactose intolerance or other situations of an enzymatic imbalance can also result in poor nutrient absorption.

Malabsorption is often at the root of poor health in our eyes, brains, and all other bodily systems. Without the nutrients from healthy foods, all the way down at the cellular level our bodies lose the ability to clear toxins from their systems. Toxin accumulation and damage is one of the biggest threats to our eyes, which is why my first and biggest dietary recommendation is always to eat more *antioxidants*.

The more antioxidants we consume, the better our chances of eliminating free radical damage in the eyes. A lot of the time, the densest quantities of antioxidants and other nutrients are found in plant parts we discard, like rinds, stalks, seeds, stems and skins. Instead of tossing them, next time add these parts to smoothies or blend them into soups or sauces as an easy way to incorporate these nutrient-dense parts of the plant.

HOW DIET AFFECTS YOUR INDIVIDUAL HEALTH

Some foods can be good for some people, but not others. People with problems metabolizing glucose should avoid foods with a high glycemic index, like bananas, because they can rapidly raise blood sugar and cause the pancreas to work overtime. Try kiwis or avocados, which have even more potassium without the side effects.

· · ·

The best way to identify where your diet is having the biggest impact on your system is through biochemistry testing. You can test the pH balance of your urine and saliva with litmus paper from the pharmacy. Stool, urine, and blood analyses will measure gastrointestinal function and bacterial balance, reveal any metabolic distress, and give a relative risk index for metabolic syndromes.

A dark field microscopic blood analysis can uncover heavy metal toxicities, a poor metabolism, endocrine imbalances, or the presence of candida. An elemental hair analysis is a simple, non-invasive screening for mineral deposits over about three months, which can reveal imbalances even before they show up in the blood. In my treatment approach, I also consider things like heredity, upbringing, trauma, lifestyle, attitudes, body chemistry, health, and disease status.

When I run biochemistry tests, I find that most of my patients are suffering from at least one of the following:

- adrenal burnout
- chronic inflammatory response
- chronic high blood sugar levels and poor glucose metabolism
- low fats in the diet

- undiagnosed sensitivities to gluten and dairy
- heavy metal toxicities

The food we eat and our body's ability to absorb those nutrients have a profound effect on the health and well-being of all systems of our bodies. ADHD and autism spectrum disorders in children, cancer, depression, Alzheimer's, Parkinson's, multiple sclerosis, and epilepsy are all connected to the nutrients we consume and our body's ability to absorb them. In optometry, poor diet or nutrient absorption translates into eyes that are more susceptible to damage.

THE RAINBOW DIET

Just as unhealthy food causes sickness, healthy food can be medicine! So much of what we need to cure ourselves of our eye problems comes through making the right eating choices.

One of the easiest ways to add more antioxidants into our diets is to follow the *rainbow diet*. By now, we've mentioned the benefits of eating a rainbow diet quite a few times, but what is it? Well, it's exactly what it sounds like – a rainbow of fruits and vegetables that span the spectrum of colors.

The strong reds, oranges, and blues in our foods are indicative of their high levels of phytochemicals, which are biological compounds found in plants. There are about 10,000 different phytochemicals and each works differently, but most have high antioxidant activity that protects against free radicals and oxidative damage. Combining a variety of different phytochemicals stimulates synergistic actions between bioactive dietary components, which is why eating from the whole rainbow provides more effective protection than sticking with one single compound.

When it comes to diet, antioxidants are the keys to fighting oxidative damage in our eyes. Oxidative damage can occur with the simple act of exercise or when your body converts food into energy, which stimulates the formation of the highly unstable molecules called free radicals. Environmental factors, such as cigarette smoke, air pollution, or even sunlight, expose your body to much higher rates of these free radicals, but all free radicals have the capacity to do the same thing – cause oxidative stress and cell damage. Oxidative stress is thought to play a role in a variety of diseases including cancer, cardiovascular disease, diabetes, Alzheimer's, Parkinson's, and eye diseases.

Within the retina, the macula has the highest metabolic needs of the whole eye, and the microcapillaries surrounding it are responsible for delivering vital nutrients. Without sufficient oxygenation and hydration in the eyes, waste easily accumulates and cuts off this flow of nutrients. Thanks to their high antioxidant content, phytochemicals improve oxidation and hydration on a cellular level, leading to increased energy production in the mitochondria and more energy in the cell to remove metabolic waste.

In cell and animal studies, antioxidant molecules have been shown to counteract oxidative stress. Most researchers believe antioxidants are behind the reduced risk of diseases for someone who consumes more fruits and vegetables. The AREDS combination of zinc and the antioxidant vitamins C and E and beta-carotene reduced the risk of advanced AMD by 25% in people with intermediate conditions or advanced in only one eye. Used without zinc, the antioxidants still reduced the risk about 17%.[14]

Red

Red colored foods may contain the phytochemicals tannins, quercetin, anthocyanins, ellagic acid, eugenol, hesperidin, but mostly the carotenoid *lycopene*. Lycopene is most abundantly found in tomatoes. Pink and orange fruits, like papaya, pink grapefruit, watermelon, and guava, also contain significant quantities of lycopene.

Some green plants, like asparagus and parsley, provide smaller amounts.

After astaxanthin, lycopene is the most potent antioxidant. Research has shown it to protect against diabetes, reduce the risk of heart disease and several cancers, including breast, lung, ovary, prostate, and stomach.[15] One study found the lycopene from tomatoes to have protective effects against prostate cancer,[16] and these effects were maintained with both raw and cooked sources,[17] making it easy to add to your diet. Lycopene also improves vascular health[18] and supports cognitive longevity in the treatment of several neuronal diseases, like Alzheimer's and depression.[19] Taking 10 mg of lycopene has also been shown to reduce pain to a similar degree as ibuprofen.[20]

Lycopene is also linked to skin health and UV protection. In one study, an oral supplement of soy isoflavones, lycopene, vitamin C, vitamin E and fish oil given to post menopausal women promoted an increased deposition of new collagen fibers in their dermis, resulting in significant wrinkle reduction.[21] Long-term consumption of lycopene may prevent skin cancer, reducing UV sun damage by 40%,[22] and providing a similar level of skin protection to SPF 1.3.[23]

Yellow and Orange

Fruits and vegetables with yellow or orange phytochemicals are high in carotenoids like beta-carotene, lutein, and zeaxanthin, and may also contain alpha-carotene, beta-cryptoxanthin, and hesperidin. Carrots, sweet potato, pumpkin, and cantaloupe are foods high in carotenoid antioxidants, and orange peppers and corn also contain significant levels of both lutein and zeaxanthin. Unlike lycopene, beta-carotene and other carotenoids convert into vitamin A once consumed, which is a vital nutrient for eye health.

Foods high in carotenoids have been shown to reduce oxidative stress and promote healthy aging.[24] Lutein and zeaxanthin are both present in high quantities in the retina and have been shown to absorb harmful blue light that enters the eyes.[25] Like other antioxidants, beta-carotene may improve memory and brain function[26] and protect against cognitive decline.[27]

Citrus fruits, like tangerines, oranges, and grapefruits, also contain high quantities of *biflavonoids*, which can be used to improve blood flow and bring down swelling.[28] One study showed citrus bioflavonoids may have hypertensive and anti-inflammatory effects in people with type 2 diabetes,[29] and oral supplementation was shown to preserve retinal sensitivity in patients with the eye condition cystoid macular edema.[30]

Green

Green foods may contain the phytochemicals epigallocatechin gallate (EGCG), glucosinolates, indoles, isoflavones, isothiocyanates, lutein, zeaxanthin, and sulforaphane. They have anti-infective and antiviral activity, and may lower the risk of cancer and reduce inflammation.[31] These phytochemicals are most abundant in vegetables like kale, cabbage, brussels sprouts, and broccoli. Some, like broccoli and spinach, also contain alpha-lipoic acid, a fatty acid and antioxidant that can cross the blood-brain barrier.

Cooked spinach, kale, romaine lettuce and parsley are some dark greens particularly high in lutein.[32] But their most protecting effects come from high levels of *glucosinolates*, sulfur-containing molecules that transform into sulforaphane. Sulforaphane has powerful anti-inflammatory effects that may prevent the development and metastasizing of cancers.[33] In studies, sulforaphane has been shown to detoxify the body of airborne pollutants,[34] and the effects of this phytochemical on oxidative stress have been shown to improve liver function.[35] A 2016 study indicated that it could help treat degeneration of the retina due to oxidative stress.[36]

Blue and Purple

The phytochemicals in purple foods can come in the form of anthocyanins, flavonoids, phenols, tannins, and resveratrol. *Anthocyanins*, found in foods like berries, red wine, and red onion, have been shown to reduce the risk of chronic disease and inflammation and improve cellular antioxidant status.[37] In addition to their antimicrobial effects, studies have shown anthocyanins to prevent cardiovascular disease, cancer, diabetes, and obesity and improve visual health.[38]

Research has also shown anthocyanins to induce ciliary muscle relaxation, promote the regeneration of the light-sensitive retinal receptor protein, rhodopsin, improve blood circulation, and may prevent the development of myopia and other optical disorders.[39]

Dark Red

Dark red nitrogen-containing pigments called *betalains* are found in some higher order fungi, but mostly in the edible form of red beetroot, prickly pear, dragon fruit, and Swiss chard.

In humans with diabetes, it was shown to improve cognitive function, glucose metabolism, and other metabolic markers.[40] Its antioxidant effects offer a promising alternative to treat diseases related to oxidative stress and inflammation,[41] including cataracts and AMD.

White and Brown

Even white and brown foods contain powerful phytochemicals like allicin, ECGC, glucosinolates, indoles, tannins, and quercetin. Onions, shallots, leeks, and garlic are all healthy white foods from the allium family that contain organosulfur compounds, like allicin and quercetin, which have anti-inflammatory properties.[42] In one study, high consumption of allium vegetables reduced the risk of developing gastric cancer.[43]

Garlic has antioxidant phytochemicals which have been indicated in reducing blood pressure and counteracting oxidative stress.[44] In one study, garlic supplementation was as effective at reducing blood pressure as the prescription drug Atenolol.[45] Studies have shown garlic to help detoxify the body of heavy metals, like lead.[46] Several studies have shown it may protect the liver cells from toxins, regulate blood sugar, reduce the risk for cardiovascular diseases, and has anti-tumor, anti-microbial, antifungal, anti-protozoal, and antiviral properties.[47]

For more healthy brown foods, try mushrooms, which contain polysaccharides, indoles, polyphenols, and carotenoids, resulting in powerful antioxidant, anti-inflammatory and anticancer effects.[48] There are more than 10,000 known types of mushrooms, but most of them contain vitamins B2, B3, B5, B9, and D, phosphorus, copper, selenium, and potassium. Studies have shown mushrooms to be capable of stimulating immune cell activity, macrophages and free radicals that attack tumor cells.[49] Other healthy white and brown foods include parsnips, white beans, soybeans, horseradish, cauliflower, bananas, lychees, potatoes, lentils, and dates.

HEALTHY FATS

Even on the rainbow diet, it's important to consume enough healthy fats for neurological health. The brain is composed of 60% fat, and as we've seen, neurological health is intrinsically tied to eye health. But many Americans lack the cholesterol and healthy fats that our nervous system needs. This is due to our belief that "low-fat" is always better, and to the medical establishment's demonization of cholesterol as a cause of arterial disease. But in reality, our bodies still need healthy fats even to make use of certain antioxidants. In a 2004 clinical trial, participants that used a fat-free dressing on their salad experienced virtually no carotenoid absorption![50]

Healthy fats are classified as monounsaturated (found in olives, olive oil, sunflower oil, avocados, almonds, pecans, cashews), or polyunsaturated (in walnuts, safflower oil, flaxseed, sunflower oil, sesame seeds, and pumpkin seeds). Unhealthy fats, on the other hand, are trans and saturated fats that come from chicken skin, fatty meats, dairy, margarine, vegetable shortening, fried foods, and candy bars. To maintain healthy cholesterol levels, get a good portion of your daily fats from foods like almonds, avocados, and fish.

HEALTHY DRINKS

Coffee

Good news for people who like their morning cup of Joe! Coffee may have health benefits beyond keeping us awake. Moderate coffee consumption has been linked with an 8% to 15% reduced risk of death, and even higher consumption levels demonstrated an even greater reduction in risk. Studies have also shown coffee to reduce the risk of cardiovascular diseases, type 2 diabetes, and cirrhosis of the liver[51] – all of which have impacts on our eye health.

Green Tea

If you're looking for a healthy drink with less caffeine than coffee, green tea may be one of the best options available. It's high in natural compounds called polyphenols that reduce inflammation. It also increases the blood's antioxidant capacity,[52] and reduces the main risk factors for cardiovascular diseases, including bad cholesterol levels.[53]

Green tea also contains a powerful antioxidant catechin called epigallocatechin-3-gallate (EGCG), which has been shown to protect cardiovascular health and have antioxidant, anti-inflammatory, anti-diabetic properties.[54] Its catechin compounds may reduce the progression of neurodegenerative disorders like Parkinson's and Alzheimer's.[55] It also contains the amino acid L-theanine, which has been shown to enhance cognitive functioning.[56] Studies show that green tea can reduce blood sugar levels and improve insulin sensitivity,[57] and green tea drinkers have a lower risk of type 2 diabetes.[58]

Coconut Water

A refreshing drink filled with natural electrolytes, like potassium, calcium and magnesium, studies have found coconut water to be even more beneficial for rehydration after exercise than water.[59] Animal studies have shown coconut water to have beneficial antioxidant effects.[60]

and it improved health markers and lowered blood sugar levels in animals with diabetes.[61]

GLOSSARY OF EYE-HEALTHY SUPER FRUITS AND VEGGIES

Asparagus:

An antioxidant powerhouse, asparagus is a great source of the antioxidant glutathione, in addition to lutein, vitamins C, E, polyphenols, and significant quantities of the flavonoids quercetin, isorhamnetin and kaempferol. It contains folic acid, which cleans the kidneys and works great as a detoxifier. Amplify its healing benefits with a light steaming.

Avocados:

Enjoy an avocado a day for a good source of omega-9 fatty acid (oleic acid), which supports liver function and reduces LDL cholesterol. Along with three grams of soluble fat, it's great for reducing inflammation of the eyes and brain. The seed is also edible and contains 20% fat as well as gut- and heart-healthy fiber. Add it to smoothies for an extra nutrient boost.

Beets:

Beets help to lower blood pressure, boost stamina, reduce inflammation, and support macula and eye health. Not only are beets a good source of fiber, they contain an array of vitamins and minerals, including folate, manganese, iron, magnesium, potassium, vitamins C and B6, and phosphorus.

Blueberries:

Their bright blue color means you can bet blueberries are high in antioxidants, which improve eye circulation. Research suggests blueberries can improve night vision and vision recovery after photobleaching[62] and like bilberry, its anthocyanins may help reverse retinal degenerative conditions.[63]

Carrots:

The beta-carotene-rich vegetable is known for eye health because of its high levels of vitamin A. Carrot seed essential oil above and below the eyes will also help oxygenate the eye tissue.

Coconut:

Coconut improves digestive health, reduces the body's inflammatory response[64] and can improve neurodegenerative diseases.[65] The high levels of lauric acid help to dissolve the lipid layer that surrounds viruses, bacteria, and pathogens, making coconut one of the best healing fats. It can also be cooked at higher temperatures than olive oil and is great for hydrating the skin after a shower.

Cordyceps:

Cordyceps are parasitic mushrooms that can be taken as a tonic to reduce respiratory disorders, improve overall oxygenation and cellular energy, and improve the immune system. You can also eat them raw, added onto salads, or in smoothies.

Corn:

Corn contains both lutein and zeaxanthin, which are essential for retinal and macular health. It also contains high amounts of lecithin, which supports healthy cell membranes throughout the body and is good for brain balance and overall blood sugar metabolism.

Endive:

A good source of fiber, folate, thiamin, niacin, pantothenic acid, pyridoxine, vitamins A and K, kaempferol and manganese. Eat two cups of endives a day for significant health benefits. They nourish the optic nerves and promote the secretion of bile to aid the liver and gallbladder.

Goji berries:

These bright red berries are clearly high in antioxidants, particularly beta-carotene, but they also contain 18 amino acids and 21 minerals.

Lime:

Lime is great for kidney and skin health. Add the pith to smoothies for valuable phytochemicals and flavonoids.

Pumpkin seeds:

Pumpkin seeds are a great source of healthy protein that are also high in fiber, vitamins E and B6, copper, manganese, zinc, and selenium. They also add good unsaturated fats to your diet, like omega-9s.

Spinach:

Not only is spinach high in carotenoids, which the body turns into vitamin A, it also contains significant levels of vitamins C, K1, folic acid, iron, and calcium. Its antioxidants will reduce oxidative stress and blood pressure levels and decrease your risk for developing cancer, and its high insoluble fiber content will help keep your digestive system healthy.

Strawberries:

These sweet treats have a low glycemic index but are high in nutrients like fiber, vitamins C and B9, manganese, and potassium. A strawberry is a powerhouse of phytochemicals, with over 25 different anthocyanins for heart health and high levels of phenolic antioxidants linked to antibacterial capabilities and a reduced risk of cancer.

GLOSSARY OF NUTRIENTS FOR EYE HEALTH

Below is a list of some of the best nutrients for eye health, along with their recommended daily allowances (RDAs). While the best way for the body to receive them is through whole foods in the diet, covering them all can be easier said than done. When you need to supplement, avoid choosing those that contain wheat, rye, barley, oats, gluten, or lactose, as well as any fillers, such as magnesium stearate, titanium dioxide, artificial colors, or hydrogenated oils.

BETA CAROTENE (RDA: 3-6 mg)

This antioxidant is the precursor to Vitamin A. Beta carotene improves macula, lens, and skin health and reduces free radical damage in the eye. It also improves night vision and reduces inflammation.

Find in: Carrots, spinach, sweet potatoes, winter squash, cantaloupe, and apricots.

GLUTATHIONE (RDA: 400-500 mg)

The "master" antioxidant helps prevent cataracts and reduces toxins, free radicals, and heavy metals in the body. Deficiencies can lead to migraines, glaucoma, cataracts, melanomas, diabetes, asthma, breast cancer, lung cancer, and Parkinson's disease.

Find in: Asparagus, potatoes, peppers, carrots, onion, broccoli, avocados, squash, spinach, garlic, tomatoes, grapefruit, apples, oranges, peaches, and bananas.

LUTEIN (RDA: 10 mg) **AND ZEAXANTHIN** (RDA: 2 mg)

Lutein and zeaxanthin to protect and strengthen the macula and the lens of the eye while also improving the immune system. They also help filter out damaging blue light, and the Age-Related Eye Disease Study (AREDS) investigated the history and risk factors of AMD and cataracts and found that high levels of lutein and zeaxanthin with zinc can lower the risk of developing AMD by up to 25%.

Find in: Egg yolks, kale, spinach, brussels sprouts, green beans, goji berries, citrus fruits, pumpkins, tomatoes, red peppers, and squash.

ASTAXANTHIN (6 mg per day)

Dr. Berne's recommendation: 6 mg per day Astaxanthin is an extremely powerful carotenoid from the microalgae. It s considered to be substantially stronger than all other well-researched antioxidants, including vitamin C, vitamin E, CoQ10, lipoic acid, and beta carotene. It also is essential in protecting the macula from blue light exposure.

MAGNESIUM (RDA: 400 mg)

Magnesium is a key mineral that helps regulate cellular energy for cardiac and skeletal muscles. It helps reduce eye twitching and spasms and protects the optic nerve and retinal tissues at the back of the eye. Magnesium can also prevent calcium build up on the lens, which can cause early onset cataracts.

Find in: Almonds, cashews, brown rice, avocados, lentils, and kidney beans.

• • •

MANGANESE (RDA: 1.8-2.3 mg)

Manganese assists with blood clotting by regulating blood sugar, metabolizing carbs, and absorbing calcium. It helps form tissues, bones, and sex hormones, and is important for fighting free radicals and optimizing nerve/brain function.

Find in: Brown rice, hazelnuts, chickpeas, spinach, pineapple, and potatoes.

OMEGA 3 FATTY ACIDS (RDA: 500-1000 mg)

Omega 3 fatty acids help lubricate the cornea, reduce eye inflammation, and protect the retina and optic nerve. They also reduce joint pain and stiffness, stabilize blood sugar, and reduce some hyperactivity symptoms.

Find in: Walnuts, egg yolks, wild-caught salmon, chia seeds, and hemp seeds.

SAFFRON (30 mg)

Dr. Berne's recommendation 30 mg per day. Saffron contains flavonoids, carotenoids, crocins and crocetin which support eye health.

SELENIUM (RDA: 50-100 micrograms)

Selenium is a trace mineral that can help prevent cataracts. It is also important for improving brain function, thyroid health, supporting a healthy immune system and fertility.

Find in: Brazil nuts, yellowfin tuna, halibut, eggs, and spinach.

TAURINE (RDA: 500-1,000 mg)

This amino acid and antioxidant can help prevent macular degeneration and glaucoma. It also helps prevent obesity, promotes glucose control, and strengthens the cardiovascular system. Studies suggest this perinatal taurine may play a role in antioxidant defenses, and deficiency in our body's natural supply can lead to oxidative stress.[66]

Find in: Salmon, tuna, shrimp, clams, eggs, beef, and lamb.

VITAMIN A (RDA: 10,000 – 25,000 IU)

Vitamin A strengthens the cornea and helps prevent dry eye, night blindness, and macular degeneration. A deficiency in vitamin A can stop the production of rhodopsin, a photopigment that the retina needs to work properly, and can result in night blindness. Vitamin A deficiency can also cause respiratory problems, dry skin, and inflammation and harms the immune system, which increases overall susceptibility to other diseases.

Find in: Eggs, carrots, squash, apricots, spinach, and kale.

VITAMIN B (RDA: 2.4-100 micrograms, depending on age)

There are three types of Vitamin B that help vision and the eyes.

- **B12**: Keeps the optic nerve healthy protecting from glaucoma, improves nerve function and supports red blood cells.
- Find in: *Lamb, cottage cheese, tuna, beef, and salmon.*
- **B6**: Reduces macular degeneration symptoms, cardiac diseases and supports immune system function. A B6 deficiency can cause blurred vision and cataract formation.

Find in: Salmon, sweet potato, bananas, and tuna.

- **B2**: Helps to reduce free radical damage and maintain healthy blood vessels. A deficiency can lead to light sensitivity, headaches, sore eyes, and cataracts.

Find in: Mushrooms, spinach, almonds, and lamb.

VITAMIN C (RDA: 200-1000 mg)

This antioxidant helps reduce free radical damage, improves mineral absorption in the lens and supports brain and immune system health.

Find in: Oranges, red peppers, kale, broccoli, grapefruit, strawberries, kiwi, and green peppers.

VITAMIN D3 (RDA: 1,000 IU)

Vitamin D3 helps prevent macular degeneration and strengthens bones and teeth. It also has anti-inflammatory properties and can help improve the immune system. Sunlight is a good source of Vitamin D3 which can prevent seasonal affective disorder and depression.

Find in: Cod liver oil, sardines, eggs, and mushrooms.

ANNATTO-E LIQUID ™ (150 mg)

Dr. Berne's recommendation 150 mg per day. This form of Vitamin E is a unique tocopherol-free, tocotrienols-only, featuring tocotrienols sourced from the annatto tree. Annatto is the richest known source of tocotrienols, containing 100% tocotrienols (90% delta- and 10% gamma-isomers) with no tocopherols. The AREDS 2 study showed Vitamin E as a beneficial nutrient in supporting eye health.

VITAMIN K (RDA: 90 mg)

This vitamin has anti-cancer properties and is important for balanced blood coagulation and increasing bone density.

Find in: Leafy green veggies, the pith of citrus fruits and wheatgrass.

ZINC (RDA: 8-11 mg)

Zinc protects the retina and lowers the risk of developing macular degeneration. It also reduces inflammation and improves circulation. Zinc improves the immune system, balances hormones, supports a healthy liver, and aids in nutrient absorption.

Find in: Kidney beans, spinach, and flax or pumpkin seeds.

CHAPTER 9
LIGHT, COLOR, AND VIBRATIONAL MEDICINE FOR HEALING THE EYES AND BODY

Traditional Western science always told us to believe without a doubt that we are finite, material beings self-contained and independent of our environment and others. Anything else, as my university professors would say, "reeks of mysticism."

But new research into light, magnetism, and other forms of energy is increasingly challenging that perspective. Technologies now allow deeper research into the dynamic energy fields that interact between and within all living things. The better we become at detecting these energies, the more repeatable patterns are emerging.

Measured on an infrared filter, for example, the human body radiates about 100 watts of energy. Cycles of the sun and the moon, light and weather patterns all impact the energy stability of our internal and external fields. The more we learn about measuring light, the more we realize how narrow of an understanding traditional Western science really is.

While not all energy is light, all light is part of the greater matrix of vibrating energies. According to Einstein's famous equation, matter and energy are two forms of the same thing, which means our bodies exist as unique energy systems within a greater energy network. That we can use these energies to heal the body is the basis for vibrational medicine.

WHAT IS LIGHT?

To understand light as a medium for healing, it's necessary for us to have a basic understanding of what light is.

Visible light comprises a small subsection of the electromagnetic spectrum. This spectrum consists of all frequencies of wave-like energy that travel through space. Oscillating electrical waves generate magnetic energy fields, which in turn generate electrical energy fields, in a continuous, self-propagating cycle. In other words, light and magnetism are intricately linked.

Electromagnetic energy travels through a stream of particles called photons. The energy in those photons determines their frequency. The only energies our eyes can perceive as light travel between 700 and 400 nanometers (nm) in wavelength.

Wavelengths shorter than 400 nm have higher frequencies and more energy to interact with matter around it, which makes them more destructive. Longer wavelengths, on the other hand, have photons with lower energy frequencies. This means they have less strength to exert onto surrounding matter (though not that they have no impact on the surrounding energy fields at all). These consist of infrared light (a radiant energy perceived as heat, but not seen), microwaves, and radio waves.

Because of their different energetic capacities, we can sit and listen to the long, low-frequency energies of radio waves for hours with no apparent effect on us, but even brief exposure to shorter frequencies can cause serious damage. For example, we already know that ultraviolet (UV) light from the sun can cause damage to our eyes. Exposure to X-rays and gamma rays, which are even shorter waves with higher frequencies, can lead to radiation sickness and cancer.

LIGHT AS MEDICINE

We've seen that since the eyes are intimately connected with other body systems, healing other body systems improves our eyes. The reverse is also true: We can leverage the power of our vision and the energy our eyes receive from light to heal other bodily systems, as well!

The Endocrine System

Once our eyes take in light, its effect is flooded through our bodies like a liquid. Almost every part of the human body is composed of fluids, making it an excellent transmitter of light energy. It travels in the form of waves, particles, or pulses, and it mirrors the energy of the fluids in our bodies. The passage of light through the eyes impacts our endocrine system, which is made up of glands that secrete hormones that regulate our emotions and behaviors.

The pupils are gates that allow light into the body, both to see and to receive fuel. Sunlight stimulates the mitochondria of our cells. Scientists have long recognized the similarities between the retinal membrane and chlorophyll molecules.[1] Both capture sunlight and convert it to a chemical impulse, but instead of using that impulse to create food, the retina converts light into an impulse and sends it to the brain to create vision.

• • •

When our eyes take in light, only 75% passes the retina, through the optic nerve and into the brain's vision centers, while the other 25% goes down the hypothalamic pathway. The hypothalamus is part of the limbic area of the brain, which supports functions of emotion, behavior, long-term memory, and smell. The hypothalamus regulates the autonomic nervous system and links it to the endocrine system through the pituitary gland.

In our brains, the pituitary gland is known as the "master gland" because of its influence on other glands. The pineal gland is connected with our third eye chakra and inner vision. The adrenal glands, located near our kidneys, are most known for producing epinephrine (adrenaline) and norepinephrine (noradrenaline) in response to stress or fear, both which stimulate our sympathetic nervous system.

Light in contact with the body's energy field stimulates the pituitary gland, which entrains the pineal, thyroid, thymus, pancreas, gonads, and adrenals. As a result, it plays a dominant role in regulating our circadian rhythms, seasonal cycles, and neuroendocrine responses. Studies by modern researchers, like Dr. George Brainard, have used this connection to define the mechanisms of light therapy that reduce the symptoms of depression, sleep problems and seasonal affective disorder.[2]

Increasingly, researchers are exploring this connection and using light therapy to regulate endocrine and nervous system function. One study found that UV radiation through the skin and eyes touches the brain and central neuroendocrine system to reset body homeostasis, suggesting its potential treatment for autoimmune and mood disorders, addiction, and obesity.[3] Research into low-level light therapy using red to near-infrared light energy has suggested the procedure might be an effective treatment for visual, neurological, and psychological conditions.[4]

Benefiting From Sunlight

According to Dr. John Ott, light is the forgotten nutrient. Just like other nutrients, our body needs it in specific quantities and meeting certain qualities. In his research, he found exposure to simulated sunlight environments reduced instances of tooth decay in children, improved classroom performance and attention, and helped students feel calmer and less nervous. When Dr. Ott broke his glasses and stopped wearing them, he accidentally healed his own arthritis at the same time, a life event that made him realize the importance of full-spectrum light passing through the unobstructed eye and reaching the pineal gland.[5]

In his 1980 book Sunlight, Dr. Zane Kime described the benefits of short exposure to trace amounts of UV light. His research showed that it enhanced the body's resistance to infections, increased cardiac output, energy levels, endurance and muscular strength while prompting the body to produce more vitamin D, which aids in the absorption of calcium and other minerals. At the same time, it decreased blood pressure and reduced resting heart rate and cholesterol.

There are three levels of UV light, and our bodies need all three types in trace amounts to support health:

- UVA (320 – 380 nm), which causes skin tanning;
- UVB (290 – 320 nm), which stimulates the production of vitamin D; and
- UVC (100 – 290 nm), which the Earth's ozone filters out before it reaches our skin.

Of course, "too much of a good thing" absolutely applies in the case of sunlight – too much exposure results in negative impacts like skin cancer and cataracts. But studies that expose animals to massive doses of UV light make it seem that you need to avoid it completely, which is not the case. In moderation, sunlight exposure can be a great benefit to the body.

Here are ways to get the right amount of sunlight needed as a nutrient for the body without subjecting yourself to potentially dangerous effects:

- Take off your sunglasses, glasses, or contacts and spend up to an hour a day outside. Put on a hat or sit in the shade if you need to, but the idea is to just bask in the natural light.

- Never look directly at the sun, especially when it's white in color, and be aware if your eyes are telling you that things are too bright to look at. Try to go out during safer periods, like before 10AM or after 4PM, when the sun's rays are less intense.

- Some Native Americans believe that looking at the pink sun during sunrise or sunset has healing properties. Even in its waning light, spending an hour in the sun will give you its benefits and may help to improve your vision.

- If you do want to wear sunglasses when you go outside, buy a neutral grey lens, which will block some, but not all, of the UV rays. I recommend the brand Environmental Lighting Concepts, which has a full spectrum sunglass with a more balanced lens that still lets in 40% of UVA and 5% of UVB rays into the eyes.

- Avoid tinted contact lenses, which cause your eyes to receive unbalanced light that they can't process without effort, resulting in light sensitivity. When you wear light-blocking lenses, most block all UV light as well as other portions of the spectrum, leading to a vision imbalance that can extend deeper into your nervous or endocrine systems.

Blue Light

No discussion on light and color is complete without a clear explanation of blue light and the risks it poses to our health. With the shortest wavelength in the visible spectrum, blue light sits right next to UV on the electromagnetic spectrum, anywhere between 380 and 500 nm.

Wavelengths between 455 and 500 nm are considered helpful. Blue light includes violet, indigo, blue and aquamarine frequencies. These color frequencies are absorbed by the retinal photopigment melanopsin and they entrain the circadian sleep and wake cycle. Morning exposure to these frequencies help you stay more alert during the day and have better sleep at night.[6]

All higher blue light frequencies between 380 and 455 can be harmful. The sun is the biggest source of this high energy visible (HEV) light, but it also comes from LED lighting and digital devices. While not as bright as the sun's HEV, these other sources still emit the same photons wavelengths and energy as hazardous light rays, but at lower intensities. However, considering how long we spend on our digital devices, the duration of exposure can accumulate to cause significant damage.

Short wavelengths are harmful because their high energy can cause photochemical damage to cells and DNA. As particles, blue light photons carry 2.5 electron-Volts (eV) or more, enough energy to create free radicals and cause oxidative stress and cell damage. Excessive HEV blue light exposure can cause visual scattering, glare, reduced contrast, and more difficulty seeing details, resulting in visual stress, eye strain and headaches.

• • •

While major outlets, like the International Organization for Standardization, have recognized the dangers of short-wavelength blue light, much of the focus is on photochemical damage from higher intensity photons over short periods of exposure, known as type II. This exposure comes primarily from sunlight. Research in the 1970s using different colored lasers on the eyes showed that short-wavelength light is more dangerous than longer wavelengths at equal intensities,[7] and blue light at 440 nm to be 20 times more dangerous than green at 533 nm.[8]

On the other hand, Type I results from low intensity blue light photons such as those from screens over long periods of exposure, and is harder to study. Not only does it require exposing children and monitoring them over their lifetimes for results, the technology and its dominance in our lives is only a recent phenomenon – so longitudinal studies are not yet available.

Through constant or repeated exposure, the low-level damage of HEV blue light accumulates throughout a life, and even without clinical trials, evidence is starting to build that Type I blue light exposure damages the eyes and disrupts sleep cycles.

Fortunately, short-wavelength light-blocking glasses seem to be effective at reducing damage. In a 2016 study, for instance, adults who wore blue-light blockers while using their digital devices two hours before bed experienced superior sleep quality.[9] Research also suggests that short-wavelength light-blocking glasses could reduce eye strain and fatigue caused by computer use[10] and improve visual function in patients with retinal diseases.[11]

COLOR THERAPY

All of this new research into light and vibration validates what many physicians have done since ancient times: Incorporating color into their healing toolkits. Egyptians built rooms inside of the pyramids as healing chambers, using sunlight filtered through colored gems in stone walls. The Greek Pythagoras is one of the first known practitioners of therapeutic healing light 2,500 years ago. Heliopolis, the Greek "City of the Sun," was famous for its healing temples that broke down sunlight into colors to treat different medical conditions.

One of the pioneers in modern color therapy, or chromotherapy, was Dr. Edwin Babbitt of New York. Among the many practical applications outlined in his book The Principles of Light and Color (1876), he explained how sunlight filtered through colored glass or water onto light-receptive autonomic nerve fibers in the skin and nerves that connect the eyes directly with the limbic system could heal the human energy field. He helped establish the New York College of Magnetics, which offered programs in chromotherapy, magnetic therapy, and psycho-emotional therapy. His work inspired scientific exploration into the field of photo-biology. [12]

Among those whom Babbitt's work inspired was Dinshah P. Ghadiali, who developed Spectro-Chrome therapy using light projected through 12 color filters and onto different body parts to heal imbalances. In 1933, The Spectro-Chrome Metry Encyclopedia elaborated his theories that our bodies are made of chemical elements as well as a balance of color waves, and that different colors can either stimulate or inhibit different organs and systems of the body. According to Ghadiali, disease occurs when there is an imbalance between those chemical elements and the color waves. Looking at the right color or shining light of that color on the body can bring balance to abnormal function or conditions within it.

In Spectro-Chrome therapy, each color has a function:

- **Green** is the equilibrator or balancer of the body
- **Lemon** (yellow-green) is for chronic conditions
- **Turquoise** (blue-green) is for acute conditions

- **Magenta** is for deeper balance
- **Scarlet** is to increase activity
- **Purple** is to decrease activity
- **Indigo** is to reduce pain or bleeding

One of the first modern practitioners to use color therapy was Dr. Harry Riley Spitler, medical doctor and optometrist whose work identified the parts of the brain connected with the autonomic nervous and endocrine systems. He found the nerve pathways of the eyes were the most direct connection to those systems and began to use light with colored lenses and gels to rebalance the nervous system and improve visual processing. In 1933, he founded the College of Syntonic Optometry. Today, Syntonic optometrists have expanded the field of research and education into Ocular Phototherapy treatment, which utilizes the different energy wavelengths of colored light to improve visual conditions and overcome diseases.

MY COLOR THERAPY PRACTICE

I first came to discover Syntonic optometry in the mid-80s when I opened my first practice, where it quickly became a keystone of my treatments. One of my first cases was a 68-year-old-woman suffering from AMD, so I followed the Syntonic guidelines and applied 20 treatments of blue-green light. Without even any vision exercises, her visual acuity improved from 20/700 to 20/150 through light therapy alone. After that, I began developing my own protocols with different lights and colors to stimulate and sensitize the photoreceptor cells in the retina.

My color therapy work began with Dr. Spitler's regimen, but linking a color with the condition alone never went deep enough to cause core visual system changes. I then started adding the methods of Dr. Jacob Liberman. At about the same time I was discovering Syntonics, Dr. Liberman developed a device called a "syntonizer" to direct different color frequencies of light into the eyes. He coined the term "color allergy" to indicate when a person is unreceptive to a particular color. He laid out a comprehensive collection of research on the healing properties of light in his book <u>Light: Medicine of the Future</u>. His research led him to develop several more phototherapy treatment devices including the Color Receptivity Trainer and the EYEPORT Vision Training System, an FDA-approved medical device for vision improvement.

In a color therapy procedure, the patient sits in a dim room looking into a color machine. I use a syntonizer, Color Receptivity Trainer and flicker device, adjusted to a speed that causes slight discomfort. As an introductory color, I start with ruby, then move up the other chakra colors to keep the energy moving; red, orange, yellow, green, blue, indigo, and violet. At each color, I tell the patient to tune into their body awareness while looking at it and I ask them to tell me what they see, feel, or remember as a result. My line of questioning helps focus their attention on what they hope to get from the session. It also keeps them in charge of their process as they uncover their deepest truths. If this process becomes too uncomfortable, the patient can choose to stop at any time.

I often use this method to treat the weaker eye in patients with lazy eye or one eye deprived of stimulation and may also use different lenses or filters over both eyes to change their processing ability. With a simpler dialogue or even a short story to accompany each color, I even apply the same approach for children, which has been successful in reducing hyperactivity, word and letter reversals, double and blurred vision, as well as poor tracking and focusing, even in children with brain injuries or multiple disabilities. Combined with vision exercises, color therapy can significantly speed up and cause breakthroughs in the process of improving your vision.

Patients who have undergone my color therapy protocols have experienced improved peripheral vision, resulting in better overall eyesight and body balance.

Children who receive the therapy end up with improved visual fields, better balance and memory, and more skills in sports and schoolwork. In my elderly patients, color therapy has been very effective for treating macular degeneration and glaucoma.

I've used color therapy on many of my patients, but I've also used it on myself in combination with my practice of yoga and meditation to connect the energy centers in my body. One of my most transforming experiences in contacting the vital energies in my own body was through incorporating the practice of yoga and meditation into my life. Before that point, my body and mind were totally split, and I relied exclusively on my intellect to process the world. Yoga helped me unite my mind-body-spirit into one system, to rejuvenate, relax, and feel in harmony for the first time in my life. My body awareness increased, and I could better experience the chakras of my body radiating to every cell, and expressed through memories, behaviors, emotions, and actions.

As our receptivity to the visible color spectrum increases, our ability to see more clearly, heal our eyesight and vision improves. Modifying the way light enters a person's eyes changes their life. By spreading the distribution of light more evenly onto the retina's 137 million photoreceptors, you increase the energy into the eyes and enhance peripheral vision, deepening eye-body relaxation and treating the whole patient – including the spirit – instead of just their symptoms.

Other Uses

In addition to improving vision, color therapy has uses in addressing other body systems. As discussed above, when color enters our eyes, the hypothalamus directs it to the brain for processing and the pineal and pituitary glands regulate hormone production in response. Within the visible spectrum, each color vibrates at a specific frequency and the frequency of each color tends to correspond to a different part of our bodies. Each body part attracts the color of its matching frequency to itself, an automatic process that helps the body stay in tune with the right frequencies, but a body part, organ or gland that falls out of its appropriate frequency can manifest as disease. While our internal frequency may vary, the color's frequency remains constant, so matching color frequencies to out-of-balance organs can restore their appropriate frequencies.

Color therapy has been used in several fields of medicine, including acupuncture, radionics, and meditation to improve mental health, reduce pain and inflammation, and improve neonatal jaundice. It can also enhance alertness, memory, reaction time, mood, and trigger relaxation. Different colors have been shown to have psychological effects on mood and behavior. Red can have an exciting effect, and yellow can boost self-esteem and creativity. Green is calming, refreshing, and harmonizing, while blue is soothing and encourages reflection. Blue can also lower blood pressure and encourage intellect, reason, and logic.[13]

In 2020, Dr. Mohab Ibrahim, associate professor of anesthesiology at the University of Arizona College of Medicine, carried out the first clinical study to evaluate green light as a potential treatment for migraines and exposure resulted in a reduction of headache days per month by an average of 60%.[14] According to Dr. Bing Liao, neurologist and Houston Methodist Hospital, green light "changes the levels of serotonin and alters the endogenous opioid system, an innate pain-relieving system found throughout the central and peripheral nervous system, gastrointestinal tract and immune system."[15]

THE ENERGY FIELD HYPOTHESIS

But going deeper than the traditional Western understanding of light provides additional pathways for healing the eyes, body, and spirit. We already know that the energy fields created by electricity and magnetism are integrally linked – but the energy field hypothesis proposes that *all* forms of energy are similarly liked. These continually moving, interrelated fields of energy are the primarily regulator of our physiology and biochemistry – even more than molecular reactions. These fields integrate and carry information throughout the body, including the eyes. Through energy coherence comes a balance between one's mind, intent, awareness, and higher self. Light, as a form of energy, is an integral component of this balance.

I believe that the planetary energetic fields and the Earth's magnetic fields affect all living things, which are interrelated and interconnected, communicating through both biological and electromagnetic fields. Both magnetic and bio-energetic fields affect our body rhythms, including heart rate, breathing, fluid resonance, nervous system, and brain waves. A static field extends above the atmosphere and shields us from solar flares and winds, created by geomagnetic fields that emulate from the Earth's core in invisible lines. When these lines flex, they influence our body rhythms, brains, nervous systems, memory and concentration, endocrine function, heart coherence and fluid bodies.

The field of chronobiology explores these energetic sensitivities to the Earth, solar, and lunar rhythms. Solar flares affect our body rhythms and increase excitability. Atmospheric magnetic fields surround us in the ionosphere like a soft plasma bubble and have a strong influence on our bodies. The Schumann Resonance between the Earth and ionosphere is a magnetic wave that vibrates at a frequency of 7.8 Hz, which matches our brains' alpha waves when in a state of well-being and harmony.

Although this may seem far-fetched to some, the research behind this idea has been growing for decades.

The positive effects of magnetism on the body have been documented since the mid-1900s. Magnetism creates restoration of cellular magnetic balance. It accelerates migration of calcium ions to help heal bones and nerve tissues. Since biomagnets are attracted to the iron in blood, they improve circulation and in turn, healing. Further, biomagnets have a positive effect on the pH balance of cells.

The American physician Andrew Bassett began to incorporate the regular use of pulsed electromagnetic field (PEMF) therapy into his practice in the 1970s. The treatment process involved pulsing magnetic fields through the body to improve circulation, cellular respiration, and nutrient intake, resulting in more balanced neurochemical levels for maintaining health.

• • •

Bassett's research led the U.S. Food and Drug Administration (FDA) to first approve use of PEMF therapy in 1979 for healing nonunion of bone. Since then, PEMF therapy and devices have received several FDA approvals, and researchers have discovered a broader range of its healing modalities. We now know that PEMF therapy has the capacity to impact virtually every single cell function, including DNA, RNA and protein synthesis, cell division and differentiation, morphogenesis, and neuroendocrine regulation.

Now, 72% of hospitals now use PEMF bone repair stimulations for fractures that are unable to heal.[16] The procedure has been shown to reduce post-operative pain,[17] to effectively treat depression,[18] and improve bone fusion and recovery from spinal surgery.[19] Even NASA has its own research program into time varying electromagnetic fields, which they believe can influence nearly all bodily tissues.[20]

During his research in the 1980s and 90s, stem cell biologist Dr. Bruce Lipton found that the outer layer of the cell processed its environment like a computer chip, which could turn genes on and off to control the behavior and physiology of the cell. Lipton's discoveries opened up the field of *epigenetics*, the study of cellular traits and the external and environmental factors that affect gene expression. In his book Biology of Belief, he described the invisible energy forces, including thoughts, that can affect our biological behavior.[21]

At about the same time, other scientists were turning to *morphogenetic* energy fields to explain why cells and bodily organs know to form their shape during development. While cells inherit fields of organization, genes don't explain the organizational form cells take. One researcher in the field of morphogenetic fields, Rupert Sheldrake, describes the term *morphic resonance* as the evolving collective memory of self-organizing patterns of a species that all members both draw upon and contribute to. Sheldrake describes these fields as underlying all mental activity and perceptions, which is why people can sense when someone else is staring at them.[22]

In 1992, Dr. Beverly Rubik coined the term "biofield" to describe the active, organizing energy field of life found within and around the body. Along with others like quantum physicist Claude Swanson, Dr. Rubik found that every biological structure receives energy both from the environment and from within the body, while also emitting its own energy into the environment. Structures in our bodies act as antennas through which we emit and receive energies from our environment and a stream of light energy or "biophotons" within.

. . .

Vibrational medicine expands on these practitioners' research with the view of humans as multi-dimensional beings made of energy fields within and surrounding them. These fields carry information for growth, development, and repair to the physical body and cells and interface with other living things. Within our genes, both molecular mechanisms and subtle energy systems govern the development of the individual cells, and researchers are discovering that these energy levels are where many disease processes begin. As light is closely connected with these other forms of energy, it follows that light, as well, impacts our wellbeing.

Through this new science, we learn to explore ourselves as more than just bodies. The intake of nutrients and oxygen does more than just fill our physical bodies. It combines with our life-force energy to fuel specialized energy-distributing systems that support the constant maintenance of our cells and organs. Eastern healing has long understood this life-force energy as *qi* or *prana*, but more Western scientists are now exploring it more deeply as their access to the technology to measure it expands.

Incredibly, there is evidence indicating that these energy fields within and surrounding us are both local and non-local, and that healing them can happen at a distance. I was writing my first book in 1994 when I first met Dr.

Hazel Parcells, 103 years old and running her newly opened retreat center. She taught me that the potential for illness can be seen in an energy field before it manifests physically, and that lower frequency disease patterns like cancer, MS, and fibromyalgia can't survive in higher vibrational environments. She also showed me that energy fields can be changed from a distance.

In her practice, Dr. Parcells would scan the body's energy patterns using a dowsing method, a pendulum, and a small sample of blood she called a "blood spot." With a special board and pendulum, she would ask questions and use the blood spot to measure the vibratory rates in the blood, glands, organs, bodily systems, as well as pH balance, cholesterol, toxicities, physiological-emotional traumas, and chakras. She would analyze this information to broadcast subtle energy frequencies of homeopathy, color, sound, gems, and crystals in a restorative process that would bring the body back into balance.

When received, these energies force people to confront the deeply held belief systems and attitudes that keep them fixed in their negative patterns. As they make the choice to raise these vibrations and accept responsibility for their own well-being, they heal both their internal diseases and external circumstances. They start to use words to describe their lives like "vibrant" and "joyful."

In vibrational medicine, emotions, behaviors, social interactions, and self-awareness can affect life-force energy. To bring the body's energy systems back into balance, vibrational healing involves various techniques, including acupuncture and acupressure, homeopathy, essential oils, sound, color, crystals, and reiki. Our life-force energy needs to be able to travel freely through the body's energy meridians, and blockages can be an underlying cause for many negative health conditions.

CHAKRAS

Such balance and transfer of energy within the body depends on a balancing of its seven main energy centers, or *chakras*. Chakras have been an important part of the practice of yoga since ancient times. In Sanskrit, the word "chakra" means "wheel." Think of them like spinning wheels of energy that integrate the cellular structures within our glands, organs, and nervous system with a flow of energy that connects the physical body to the spiritual. The position of each chakra relates directly to both a major nerve plexus and endocrine gland, and each has a unique physiological and psychospiritual meaning in the body.

The chakras are responsible for our patterns in behavior, attitudes, thoughts, and beliefs as well as physiological problems in the nervous system. To function at their best, their flow needs to stay open and unblocked. Opening your chakras helps reconnect the organs, glands, and nervous centers of the body, and doing this through light therapy expands your inner vision. To be in balance, their position in the body should be aligned in a vertical column from the base of the spine to the top of the head.

The frequency of light and energy for each chakra also matches a color in the visible energy spectrum – and many of them have a correlation with certain types of eye problems.

The Root Chakra: RED

This chakra sits at the base of the spine right at the coccyx bone. It interacts with the colon and small intestine and is involved with release of digestive materials. Within this chakra, we store our intense fears and the will to live. This is a place of primal energy. Getting your root chakra in line helps to keep the rest in line. People with myopia tend to hold blocked unconscious energy concerning survival issues in this chakra.

The Sacral Chakra: ORANGE

Located halfway between the navel and genitals, the sacral chakra sits near the spleen and interacts with the gonads, reproductive organs, bladder, large and small intestines, and the lumbar vertebrae. This chakra houses our passion, vibrancy, and sensuality, both masculine and feminine energies combined. Blocks in this chakra manifest as pain, grief, and shame, and can often indicate unresolved histories of sexual abuse. In the eyes, this manifests as one eye seeing better than the other, or significant myopia or hyperopia.

The Solar Plexus: YELLOW

Sitting right at the tip of the sternum, this chakra falls between the base of the ribs and the navel. It provides energy to the stomach, gallbladder, spleen, liver and pancreas. The solar plexus is the center of the will, intellectual power and ego. Its free flow determines your access to personal power. Blockages here can indicate inner anger, feeling like a victim or disempowerment. In vision, people with a blocked solar plexus usually have hyperopia or myopia over +/− 3.00 diopters, taking away their internal power and putting it all into their lenses, outside of themselves. As a result, they feel deep insecurities about seeing, trusting, and intimacy.

The Heart Center: GREEN

Just like it sounds, this chakra sits directly over the heart and thymus gland and supports the heart, lungs, breasts, and circulatory system. It represents our expressions of love and compassion, goodwill, forgiveness, nurturance, and detachment. Developing a strong sense of self-love is one of the most important keys to opening this chakra. Blockages in this chakra manifest in the eyes as someone who sees through a filter of fear, either pushing the world away or pulling it in very close, which can often result in glaucoma.

The Throat Center: BLUE

This chakra is at the middle of the throat, right over the thyroid and larynx. It influences the parathyroid and thyroid glands, vocal cords, mouth, trachea, and cervical vertebrae. It also interacts with the vagus nerve, which connects the heart and brainstem through the neck and regulates the parasympathetic nervous system. This chakra reflects our communication and self-expression. Blockages can lead a person to hide their true inner feelings or needs. Fear closes down the chakra and creates a narrow view, which is why in the eyes, this often manifests as myopia. Because of its frequency, turquoise is a very helpful in color therapy to open the throat chakra and reduce myopia.

The Third Eye: INDIGO

Situated right in the middle of our forehead, the third eye influences our sinuses, eyes, pineal organ, and pituitary gland. When open, you can see your inner vision or destiny and better connect to your own spirit. The more clearly we see our own spirit, the better we express our true selves to the world. Our intuition becomes one with universal consciousness. Energy blockages, on the other hand, result in endocrine imbalances, sinus problems, and mental confusion. In vision, a blockage in the third eye can result in the two external eyes being unable to work together – an underlying cause of strabismus, amblyopia, or diplopia.

The Crown Chakra: PURPLE

This chakra sits at the top of the head and influences the nervous system, cerebral cortex, and integration between the right and left hemispheres of the brain. It represents one's higher states of awareness and a deep spiritual knowledge of the self and outer world. Open, this chakra represents a total alignment of the body, mind, and spirit within and without. You may experience a state of connection with everything in the universe and your eyes may see visible manifestations of energy auras in the world around them. Closed, however, and the mind, body, and spirit are in confusion. This could manifest as dyslexia or even serious forms of mental illness.

The Body's Energy

A blockage in any of your chakras cuts off the body from its life-force energy, which can manifest as negative conditions on the body, mind, and spirit. By using the right frequencies to address the particular chakra, however, light and color therapy can help to keep them open and in free movement.

In 2014, I conducted the Esalen Color Therapy Study on 20 subjects treated with the rainbow color method using red, orange, yellow, green, blue, violet, and magenta. At the outset of the study, I measured each person's energy field, acupuncture meridians, and chakras. I adjusted the brightness of each color to a comfortable level and had the participants look through each one for 2 minutes, telling them to imagine living in a color dome or bathing in the color until the whole body fills up with it. We repeated this two times a day over seven days and on day 8, I took the same measurements and found an increase in energy field illumination and size, as well as chakra alignment by 80%.

Mainstream science can detect these energy readings using an EKG for heart waves or EEG for brain waves, but other techniques include thermography and electrodermal measurements. In the 1940s, electrician Seymour Kirlian developed a type of photography by running low voltage currents through living things and observing and measuring the patterns created by the discharge of energy. Through Kirlian photography, we can identify compressions, traumas, toxicities, and the influence of electronics in the body.

For my work, I mostly use a Gas Discharge Visualization (GDV) camera, which is a biomedical instrument invented by Russian biophysicist Konstantin Korotkov. Extensive studies starting in 1997 demonstrated that GDV gives quantifiable, reproducible, and consistent energy readings similar to Kirlian photographs. The same person measured three days in a row would have identical energy patterns each time, called an "energetic signature," and this method is an accepted diagnostic technique for the Russian Academy of Science.

These devices bridge our understanding of the unseen world with the physical by capturing images of the living energy fields around people, animals, plants, water, essential oils, light, sound, crystals, and more. They measure the levels of photons, meridians, and chakras within the body and the external transfers they make outside of it. Adding subtle energies like light, sound, or essential oils to the body results in measurable improvements in GDV readings, for example, whereas the addition of synthetic products, like pharmaceuticals, causes a measurable detriment.

To read your energy levels, I would have you place your fingertips, the endpoints of major acupuncture meridians that correlate with health and disease, on a highly-charged glass plate. The electrical charge induces the discharge of energy from each finger and the GDV camera captures, analyzes and reproduces it in a sequence of light patterns. From these patterns, it extracts data to plot the energy associated with the various organs, tissues, and glands on each side of your body. These results give me a lot of insight into the traumas, acute and chronic health problems from physical, emotional, psychological, and spiritual perspectives of a person, as well as the size and alignment of their chakras. This first step allows me to better suggest the next steps for treatment.

According to Professor Fritz-Albert Popp, a cell in optimal health will respond to all colors of the visible spectrum equally. By shining the right color light onto the right body part, this can re-awaken memories, emotions or experiences stored there that were previously too painful to acknowledge. Habitual triggers inside ourselves cause certain colors to make us feel uncomfortable, and this reaction helps identify those triggers so they can be dissolved. By overcoming these emotions and sensations that block our energy flow, we experience more freedom in our awareness and vision.

When light fills up the body, patients can more clearly see their inner vision, discover core misperceptions about their awareness and behavior and release that blocked energy. Light opens up more space within so that old patterns and conditioning, even at a cellular vibrational level, can more easily be reprogrammed. As light frees people from their conditioning, they learn to trust their own intuition and creativity.

This is why color therapy sometimes brings up old, stored memories, emotions, and perceptions. The body is purging them as a way of detoxification, and these responses to each color can indicate which chakra is out of balance. In combination with the help of a trained therapist, a light therapy practitioner can help a patient release their old patterns and make way for new ones. Just like the sensations of the treatment itself, it may start with a feeling of heat or movement of energy, but this soon makes way for a sense of peace and openness.

The eyes receive and radiate light. The more we can take in, the more we can radiate our true self. In our awareness, there is an outer vision that sees the world and an inner vision of how we see ourselves and the fastest and most direct way to heal our outer vision is to heal the inner vision first. When light fills up the dark places of our inner vision, we can see inside of ourselves without denial, and the clearer our inner vision becomes. Light is a clear mirror in which we can see our inner vision at a deeper level.

The movement of our energy both shapes and is shaped by our environment. Like sensitive antennas sending out and receiving low-level starlight, each atom in our skin emits 2000 photons per second. If we all gave off love, compassion, and gratitude, it would offset the state of incoherence and stress currently dominating our society.

Our vision is our guidance system and disease in the eyes tells us that something is out of balance. Physical discomfort is usually in direct proportion to our resistance to change. Ignoring the signs of imbalance lets the condition manifest and build strength, resulting in greater physical discomfort. Choosing health, on the other hand, is choosing to live in a more authentic way not covering up symptoms, but focusing instead on healing the underlying causes.

ABOUT THE AUTHOR

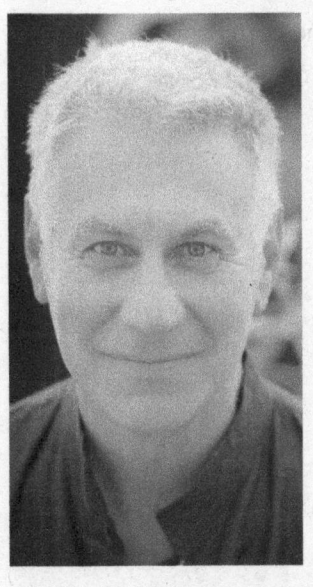

Dr Sam Berne has been in private practice for over 25 years, where he works with patients to improve their vision and overall wellness through holistic methods. He holds a Bachelor of Science from Pennsylvania State University, Doctor of Optometry from Pennsylvania College and did his postdoctoral work at the Gesell Institute in collaboration with Yale University. He has been awarded The Special Awards for Service from the Behavioral Optometrists in Mexico for his innovative and holistic work with children.

His protocols take a proactive, rather than reactive, approach to health and wellness. He understands and treats the body as one integrated system, rather than a collection of independent organs, in order to identify and address the root causes of disease. His whole health protocols improve vision and wellness by healing the mind-body-spirit through nutritional protocols, vision therapy, and self-care techniques. This views each person as genetically and biochemically unique and enables the individual to make lifelong improvements to their well-being.

Find out more at:
https://www.drsamberne.com/about/

NOTES

1. FLOATERS

1. U.S. Food and Drug Administration. (n.d.). *Dental Amalgam Fillings*. Retrieved July 29, 2021 from https://www.fda.gov/medical-devices/dental-devices/dental-amalgam-fillings
2. Kim, J., Lee, J., Kim, H., Kim, K. & Kim, H. (2019). Possible Effects of Radiofrequency Electromagnetic Field Exposure on Central Nerve System. *Biomolecules & Therapuetics*, 27(3), 265-275. https://doi.org/0.4062/biomolther.2018.152
3. Webb, B. F., Webb, J. R., Schroeder, M. C., & North, C. S. (2013). Prevalence of vitreous floaters in a community sample of smartphone users. *International Journal of Ophthalmology*, 6(3), 402–405. https://doi.org/10.3980/j.issn.2222-3959.2013.03.27
4. Yonemoto, J., Ideta H., Sasaki K., Tanaka S., Hirose A., Oka C. (1994). The age of onset of posterior vitreous detachment. *Graefes Archives for Clinical and Experimental Ophthalmology*, 232(2), 67-70. https://doi.org/10.1007/BF00171665
5. Phulke, S., Kaushik, S., Kaur, S., & Pandav, S. S. (2017). Steroid-induced Glaucoma: An Avoidable Irreversible Blindness. *Journal of current glaucoma practice*, 11(2), 67–72. https://doi.org/10.5005/jp-journals-l0028-1226
6. Drugs.com. (2020, July 9). *Elavil*. https://www.drugs.com/elavil.html
7. Dooley, M., & McMahon, S. W. (2020). A Comprehensive Review of Mold Research Literature from 2011 – 2018. *Internal Medicine Review*. https://internalmedicinereview.org/index.php/imr/article/view/836.
8. Thomas, N. (n.d.). Understanding Chronic Inflammatory Response Syndrome (CIRS). Survivingmold.com. https://www.survivingmold.com/docs/UNDERSTANDING_CIRS_ED ITV2A.PDF.
9. GeneCards. (n.d.) *HLA-DRA Gene – Major Histocompatibility Complex, Class II, DR Alpha*. https://www.genecards.org/cgi-

NOTES

bin/carddisp.pl?gene=HLA-DRA

LIFESTYLE CHANGES TO ADDRESS FLOATERS

1. Fitzpatrick, R.E., & Rostan, E.F. (2002). Double-blind, half-face study comparing topical vitamin C and vehicle for rejuvenation of photodamage. *Dermatologic Surgery, 28*(3), 231-6. https://doi.org/10.1046/j.1524-4725.2002.01129.x
2. Alanazi, S. A., El-Hiti, G. A., Al-Baloud, A. A., Alfarhan, M. I., Al-Shahrani, A., Albakri, A. A., Alqahtani, S., & Masmali, A. M. (2019). Effects of short-term oral vitamin A supplementation on the ocular tear film in patients with dry eye. *Clinical ophthalmology, 2019*(13), 599–604. https://doi.org/10.2147/OPTH.S198349
3. Jiang Y., Wu, S., Shu, X. Xiang, Y., Ji, B., Milne, G., Cai, Q., Zhang, X., Gao, Y., Zheng, W., & Yang, G. (2014) Cruciferous vegetable intake is inversely correlated with circulating levels of proinflammatory markers in women. *Journal of the Academy of Nutrition and Dietetics, 114*(5):700-708.E2. https://doi.org/10.1016/j.jand.2013.12.019
4. Office of Dietary Supplements. (2021, March). *Vitamin C: Fact Sheet for Health Professionals.* US Department of Health and Human Services, National Institutes of Health. https://ods.od.nih.gov/factsheets/VitaminC-HealthProfessional/
5. Ibid.
6. Gasparrini, M., Forbes-Hernandez, T. Y., Giampieri, F., Afrin, S., Alvarez-Suarez, J. M., Mazzoni, L., Mezzetti, B., Quiles, J. L., & Battino, M. (2017). Anti-inflammatory effect of strawberry extract against LPS-induced stress in RAW 264.7 macrophages. *Food and chemical toxicology, 102*(4), 1–10, 102. https://doi.org/10.1016/j.fct.2017.01.018
7. Basu, A., Fu, D. X., Wilkinson, M., Simmons, B., Wu, M., Betts, N. M., Du, M., & Lyons, T. J. (2010). Strawberries decrease atherosclerotic markers in subjects with metabolic syndrome. *Nutrition Research 30*(7), 462–469. https://doi.org/10.1016/j.nutres.2010.06.016

NOTES

8. Kim, J, Lee, J., Kim, H., Kim, K, Kim, H. (2019). Possible Effects of Radiofrequency Electromagnetic Field Exposure on Central Nerve System. *Biomolecules and Therapeutics*, 27(3), 265-275. https://doi.org/10.4062/biomolther.2018.152
9. Song, K.C., et al. (2012). Processed Panax ginseng, Sun Ginseng Increases Type I Collagen by Regulating MMP-1 and TIMP-1 Expression in Human Dermal Fibroblasts. *Journal of Ginseng Research*. 36(1), 61–67. https://doi.org/10.5142/jgr.2012.36.1.61
10. Nutritionvalue.org. (n.d.). "Cilantro, raw." https://www.nutritionvalue.org/Cilantro%2C_raw_75109550_nutritional_value.html?size=100+g
11. Thomas, N. V., & Kim, S. K. (2013). Beneficial effects of marine algal compounds in cosmeceuticals. *Marine Drugs*, 11(1), 146–164. https://doi.org/10.3390/md11010146
12. Liu, H., et al. (2010). Fructose Induces Transketolase Flux to Promote Pancreatic Cancer Growth. *Cancer Research*, 70(15), 6368-6376. https://cancerres.aacrjournals.org/content/70/15/6368
13. Dabrowiecki, A., Villalobos, A., & Krupinski, E.A. (2020). Impact of blue light filtering glasses on computer vision syndrome in radiology residents: a pilot study. *Journal of Medical Imaging*, 7(2). https://doi.org/10.1117/1.JMI.7.2.022402

2. CATARACTS

1. World Health Organization (2019). *World Report on Vision*. https://www.who.int/publications/i/item/9789241516570
2. National Eye Institute. (n.d). "Cataract Data and Statistics." U.S. Department of Health and Human Services, National Institutes of Health. https://www.nei.nih.gov/learn-about-eye-health/resources-for-health-educators/eye-health-data-and-statistics/cataract-data-and-statistics
3. Kellogg Eye Center. (n.d.). *Cataracts*. University of Michigan Health. http://www.kellogg.umich.edu/patientcare/conditions/cataract.html
4. Sabhapandit, S. (2020, January 7). *Cortical cataracts symptoms, causes and treatment*. Neoretina Eyecare Institute. https://neoretina.com/blog/cortical-cataracts-symptoms-causes-and-treatment/

NOTES

5. Stanford Children's Health. (n.d.). *Cataracts in Children*. https://www.stanfordchildrens.org/en/topic/default?id=cataracts-in-children-90-P02105

6. Kiziltoprak, H., Tekin, K., Inanc, M., & Goker, Y. S. (2019). Cataract in diabetes mellitus. *World Journal of Diabetes, 10*(3), 140–153. https://doi.org/10.4239/wjd.v10.i3.140

7. Drake, V. (2017, November). *Micronutrient Inadequacies in the US Population: an Overview*. Oregon State University, Linus Pauling Institute. https://lpi.oregonstate.edu/mic/micronutrient-inadequacies/overview

8. Mares-Perlman, J. A., Lyle, B. J., Klein, R., Fisher, A. I., Brady, W. E., VandenLangenberg, G. M., Trabulsi, J. N., & Palta, M. (2000). Vitamin supplement use and incident cataracts in a population-based study. *Archives of Ophthalmology, 118*(11), 1556–1563. https://doi.org/10.1001/archopht.118.11.1556

9. Junqing An, et al. (2021). Western-style diet impedes colonization and clearance of Citrobacter rodentium. *Plos Pathogens*. https://doi.org/10.1371/journal.ppat.1009497

10. National Eye Institute. (2014). *New Research Sheds Light on How UV Rays May Contribute to Cataracts*. U.S. Department of Health and Human Services, National Institutes of Health. https://www.nei.nih.gov/about/news-and-events/news/new-research-sheds-light-how-uv-rays-may-contribute-cataract

11. Ouyang X, et al. (2020). Mechanisms of blue light-induced eye hazard and protective measures: a review. *Biomedicine and Pharmacotherapy, (130)*110577. https://doi.org/10.1016/j.biopha.2020.110577

12. Centers for Disease Control and Prevention. (2018). *State Indicator Report on Fruits and Vegetables*. https://www.cdc.gov/nutrition/data-statistics/2018-state-indicator-report-fruits-vegetables.html

13. Wallace T.C., et al. (2020). Fruits, vegetables, and health: A comprehensive narrative, umbrella review of the science and recommendations for enhanced public policy to improve intake. *Critical Reviews in Food Science and Nutrition, 60*(13) https://doi.org/10.1080/10408398.2019.1632258

14. Rathbun, W. B., Nagasawa, H. T., & Killen, C. E. (1996). Prevention of naphthalene-induced cataract and hepatic glutathione loss by the L-cysteine prodrugs, MTCA and PTCA. *Experimental Eye Research, 62*(4), 433–441. https://doi.org/10.1006/exer.1996.0048

15. Weschawalit, S., Thongthip, S., Phutrakool, P., & Asawanonda, P. (2017). Glutathione and its antiaging and antimelanogenic effects. *Clinical, Cosmetic and Investigational Dermatology*. 2017(10), 147–153. https://doi.org/10.2147/CCID.S128339
16. Patrick, L. (2002). Mercury toxicity and antioxidants: Part 1: role of glutathione and alpha-lipoic acid in the treatment of mercury toxicity. *Alternative Medicine Review*. 7(6), 456-71. https://pubmed.ncbi.nlm.nih.gov/12495372/
17. Schmeling, M., Gaynes, B., & Tidow-Kebritchi, S. (2014). Heavy metal analysis in lens and aqueous humor of cataract patients by total reflection X-ray fluorescence spectrometry. *Powder Diffraction*, 29(2), 155-158. https://doi.org/10.1017/S0885715614000281
18. Richie, J.P., et al. (2015). Randomized controlled trial of oral glutathione supplementation on body stores of glutathione. *European Journal of Nutrition*, 54(2), 251-63. https://doi.org/10.1007/s00394-014-0706-z
19. Nimni, M.E., Han, B. & Cordoba, F. (2007). Are we getting enough sulfur in our diet?. *Nutrition and Metabolism*, 4(24). https://doi.org/10.1186/1743-7075-4-24
20. Robertson, J.M., et al. (1991). "A possible role for vitamins C and E in cataract prevention." *American Journal of Clinical Nutrition*, 53(1). https://doi.org/10.1093/ajcn/53.1.346S
21. Jacques PF, et al. (2001). Long-term nutrient intake and early age-related nuclear lens opacities. *Archives of Ophthalmology*, 119(7), 1009-19. https://doi.org/10.1001/archopht.119.7.1009
22. Yonova-Doing, Ekaterina, et al. (2016). Genetic and Dietary Factors Influencing the Progression of Nuclear Cataract. *Ophthalmology*, 123(6), 1237-1244. https://www.aaojournal.org/article/S0161-6420(16)00114-7/fulltext
23. Robertson JM, et al. (1991). A possible role for vitamins C and E in cataract prevention. *American Journal of Clinical Nutrition*, 53(1), 346S-351S. https://doi.org/10.1093/ajcn/53.1.346S
24. Abdul Nasir, N. A., et al. (2014). Effects of topically applied tocotrienol on cataractogenesis and lens redox status in galactosemic rats. *Molecular Vision*, 20, 822–835. https://pubmed.ncbi.nlm.nih.gov/24940038/
25. Kuzniarz M., et al. (2001). Use of vitamin supplements and cataract: the Blue Mountains Eye Study. *American Journal of*

NOTES

      Ophthalmology, *132*(1), 19-26. https://doi.org/10.1016/s0002-9394(01)00922-9

26. Wang A., et al. (2014). Association of vitamin A and β-carotene with risk for age-related cataract: a meta-analysis. *Nutrition*, *30*(10), 1113-21. https://doi.org/10.1016/j.nut.2014.02.025
27. Christen W.G., et al. (2003) A Randomized Trial of Beta Carotene and Age-Related Cataract in US Physicians." *Archives of Ophthalmology*, *121*(3), 372–378. https://doi.org/10.1001/archopht.121.3.372
28. Yeum K.J., et al. (1995). Measurement of carotenoids, retinoids, and tocopherols in human lenses. *Investigative Ophthalmology & Visual Science*, *36*(13), 2756-61. https://pubmed.ncbi.nlm.nih.gov/7499098/
29. Mazzotta, Cosimo, et al. (2014). Riboflavin and the Cornea and Implications for Cataracts. In V. Preedy (Ed.), *Handbook of Nutrition, Diet and the Eye* (pp 123-130). Academic Press. https://doi.org/10.1016/B978-0-12-401717-7.00013-7
30. Rao, P., et al. (2015). The Relationship Between Serum 25-Hydroxyvitamin D Levels and Nuclear Cataract in the Carotenoid Age-Related Eye Study (CAREDS), an Ancillary Study of the Women's Health Initiative. *Investigative Ophthalmology & Visual Science*, *56*(8), 4221–4230. https://doi.org/10.1167/iovs.15-16835
31. Lee S.H., et al. (2012). Comparative ocular microbial communities in humans with and without blepharitis. *Investigative Ophthalmology & Visual Science*, *53*(9), 5585-93. https://doi.org/10.1167/iovs.12-9922
32. Pineau, A., et al. (1992). A Study of Chromium in Human Cataractous Lenses and Whole Blood of Diabetics, Senile and Normal Population. *Biological Trace Element Research*, *32*, 133-138. https://www.academia.edu/12493308/A_study_of_chromium_in_human_cataractous_lenses_and_whole_blood_of_diabetics_senile_and_normal_population
33. Post M., et al. (2018). Serum selenium levels are associated with age-related cataract. *Annals of Agricultural and Environmental Medicine*, *25*(3), 443-448. https://doi.org/10.26444/aaem/90886
34. Zhu, Xiangjia, et al. (2014). Selenium Supplementation and Cataract. In V. Preedy (Ed.) *Handbook of Nutrition, Diet and the Eye* (pp 123-130). Academic Press. https://doi.org/10.1016/B978-0-12-401717-7.00016-2

35. Agarwal R., et al. (2013). Mechanisms of cataractogenesis in the presence of magnesium deficiency. *Magnesium Research, 26*(1), 2-8. https://doi.org/10.1684/mrh.2013.0336
36. Grahn B.H., et al. Zinc and the eye. *Journal of the American College of Nutrition, 20*(2),106-18. https://doi.org/10.1080/07315724.2001.10719022
37. Barman S., et al. (2019) Supplementation Ameliorates Diabetic Cataract Through Modulation of Crystallin Proteins and Polyol Pathway in Experimental Rats. *Biological Trace Elements Research, 187*(1), 212-223. https://doi.org/10.1007/s12011-018-1373-3
38. Vimont, C. (2020, October 15). *The Benefits of Fish Oil for Dry Eye*. American Academy of Ophthalmology. https://www.aao.org/eye-health/tips-prevention/does-fish-oil-help-dry-eye
39. Martínez-Lapiscina E.H., et al. (2010) Consumo de ácidos grasos e incidencia de cataratas: estudio de la cohorte Seguimiento Universidad de Navarra [Dietary fat intake and incidence of cataracts: The SUN Prospective study in the cohort of Navarra, Spain]. *Medicina Clínica, 134*(5), 194-201. https://doi.org/10.1016/j.medcli.2009.09.041
40. Wu K.L., et al. (2008). Effects of ginger on gastric emptying and motility in healthy humans. *European Journal of Gastroenterology and Hepatology, 20*(5), 436-40. https://doi.org/10.1097/MEG.0b013e3282f4b224
41. Hendrick, B. (2011, April 20). *Vegetarians May Have Lower Risk of Cataracts*. WebMD. https://www.webmd.com/eye-health/cataracts/news/20110420/vegetarians-may-have-lower-risk-of-cataracts
42. Dubois V.D., & Bastawrous A. N-acetylcarnosine (NAC) drops for age-related cataract. *The Cochrane Database of Systemic Reviews, 2017*(2), 1-14. https://doi.org/10.1002/14651858.CD009493.pub2
43. Taheri, S., et al. (2020). Effect of intensive lifestyle intervention on bodyweight and glycaemia in early type 2 diabetes (DIADEM-I): an open-label, parallel-group, randomised controlled trial. *The Lancet, 8*(6). https://www.thelancet.com/journals/landia/article/PIIS2213-8587(20)30117-0/fulltext
44. Rosenfarb, A. (2012). Researching Retinitis Pigmentosa (Night Blindness) with Acupuncture and Chinese Medicine. *Oriental Medicine*. https://issuu.com/pacificcollege/docs/om_spr12_web

NOTES

45. Namazi M., et al. (2014). Aromatherapy with citrus aurantium oil and anxiety during the first stage of labor. *Iran Red Crescent Medical Journal. 16*(6), e18371. https://doi.org/10.5812/ircmj.18371
46. Khodabakhsh P., et al. (2015). Analgesic and anti-inflammatory activities of Citrus aurantium L. blossoms essential oil (neroli): involvement of the nitric oxide/cyclic-guanosine monophosphate pathway. *Journal of Natural Medicine, 69*(3), 324-31. https://doi.org/10.1007/s11418-015-0896-6
47. Cho, M.Y., et al. (2013). Effects of aromatherapy on the anxiety, vital signs, and sleep quality of percutaneous coronary intervention patients in intensive care units. *Evidence-based Complementary and Alternative Medicine,* 2013. https://doi.org/10.1155/2013/381381
48. Hwang, J.H. (2006). The effects of the inhalation method using essential oils on blood pressure and stress responses of clients with essential hypertension. *Journal of Korean Academy of Nursing, 36*(7), 1123-34. https://doi.org10.4040/jkan.2006.36.7.1123
49. Kim JH, et al. (2019). Possible Effects of Radiofrequency Electromagnetic Field Exposure on Central Nerve System. *Biomolecules and Therapeutics,* 27(3), 265-275. https://doi.org/10.4062/biomolther.2018.152

3. MACULAR DEGENERATION

1. BrightFocus Foundation. (2019, January 5). *Age-Related Macular Degeneration: Facts & Figures.* https://www.brightfocus.org/macular/article/age-related-macular-facts-figures
2. Pilgrim, M., et al. (2017). Subretinal Pigment Epithelial Deposition of Drusen Components Including Hydroxyapatite in a Primary Cell Culture Model. *Investigative Ophthalmology & Visual Science, 58*(2), 708-719. https://doi.org/10.1167/iovs.16-21060
3. Pizzino, G., et al. (2017). Oxidative Stress: Harms and Benefits for Human Health. *Oxidative Medicine and Cellular Longevity,* 2017. https://www.hindawi.com/journals/omcl/2017/8416763/
4. Chalam K.V., et al. (2011). A review: role of ultraviolet radiation in age-related macular degeneration. *Eye Contact Lens: Science and*

Clinical Practice, 37(4), 225-32. https://doi.org/10.1097/ICL.0b013e31821fbd3e

5. Roberts, J.E. (2011). Ultraviolet radiation as a risk factor for cataract and macular degeneration. Eye & Contact Lens, 37(4), 246-9. https://doi.org/10.1097/ICL.0b013e31821cbcc9
6. Carnevale, R., et al. (2018, November 5). Effects of Smoking on Oxidative Stress and Vascular Function. in Smoking Prevention and Cessation. IntechOpen. https://www.intechopen.com/chapters/61774.
7. Khan J.C., et al, (2006). Genetic Factors in AMD Study. Smoking and age related macular degeneration: the number of pack years of cigarette smoking is a major determinant of risk for both geographic atrophy and choroidal neovascularisation. *The British Journal of Ophthalmology*, 90(1), 75-80. https://doi.org/10.1136/bjo.2005.073643
8. Wisconsin Department of Health Services. (2015, December 21). *Medication and other agents that Increase Sensitivity to Light*. https://www.dhs.wisconsin.gov/radiation/medications.htm.
9. Ibid.
10. Ibid.
11. Ibid.
12. Ibid.
13. eHealthMe. (2021, May 23). *Clonidine and Macular degeneration – a phase IV clinical study of FDA data*. https://www.ehealthme.com/ds/clonidine/macular-degeneration/.
14. Geamănu Pancă, A., et al. (2014). Retinal toxicity associated with chronic exposure to hydroxychloroquine and its ocular screening. Review. *Journal of Medicine and Life*, 7(3), 322–326. https://www.ncbi.nlm.nih.gov/pmc/articles/PMC4233433/
15. Edwards, D.R., et al. (2010). Inverse association of female hormone replacement therapy with age-related macular degeneration and interactions with ARMS2 polymorphisms. *Investigative Ophthalmology & Visual Science*, 51(4), 1873–1879. https://doi.org/10.1167/iovs.09-4000
16. van Leeuwen, R., et al. (2004). Cholesterol and age-related macular degeneration: is there a link? *American Journal of Ophthalmology*, 137(4),750-752. https://doi.org/10.1016/j.ajo.2003.09.015
17. Colijn, J., et al. (2019). Increased High-Density Lipoprotein Levels Associated with Age-Related Macular Degeneration: Evidence

NOTES

from the EYE-RISK and European Eye Epidemiology Consortia. *Ophthalmology*, 126(3), 393–406. https://doi.org/10.1016/j.ophtha.2018.09.045

18. National Eye Institute. (n.d). *AREDS/AREDS2 Frequently Asked Questions*. National Institutes of Health. https://www.nei.nih.gov/research/clinical-trials/age-related-eye-disease-studies-aredsareds2/aredsareds2-frequently-asked-questions
19. Godman, Heidi. (2019, October 4). *Macular Degeneration Surgery: How to Prepare, What Happens and Risks*. U.S. News. https://health.usnews.com/conditions/eye-disease/macular-degeneration/articles/macular-degeneration-surgery-how-to-prepare.
20. Ibid
21. Spooner K., et al. (2021). Long-term Anti-Vascular Endothelial Growth Factor Treatment for Neovascular Age-Related Macular Degeneration: The LATAR Study: Report 1: Ten-Year, Real-World Outcomes. *Ophthalmology Retina*, 5(6), 511-518. https://doi.org/10.1016/j.oret.2020.09.019
22. Reid, C. A., et al. (2018). Development of an inducible anti-VEGF rAAV gene therapy strategy for the treatment of wet AMD. *Scientific Reports*, 8(1), Article 11763. https://doi.org/10.1038/s41598-018-29726-7
23. Age Related Eye Diseases. (n.d.). *Age Related Eye Disease Studies (AREDS)*. https://areds.org/
24. Ramakrishna, M., & Suresh V. (2013). Apple peels – a versatile biomass for water purification? *ACS Applied Materials & Interfaces*, 5(1), 4443-4449. https://doi.org/10.1021/am400901e
25. Kooti, W., & Nahid D. A Review of the Antioxidant Activity of Cerly (Apium graveolens L). *Journal of Evidence-Based Integrative Medicine*, 22(4), 1029-1034. https://journals.sagepub.com/doi/10.1177/2156587217717415?url_ver=Z39.88-2003&rfr_id=ori%3Arid%3Acrossref.org&rfr_dat=cr_pub++0pubmed&.
26. El-Shinnawy N.A. (2015). The therapeutic applications of celery oil seed extract on the plasticizer di(2-ethylhexyl) phthalate toxicity. *Toxicology and Industrial Health*, 31(4), 355-66. https://doi.org/10.1177/0748233713475515
27. Merle B.M.J., et al. (2019). Mediterranean Diet and Incidence of Advanced Age-Related Macular Degeneration: The EYE-RISK Consortium. *Ophthalmology*, 126(3), 381-390. https://doi.org/10.1016/j.ophtha.2018.08.006

28. Sandberg, M., et al. (2014). The Relationship of Central Foveal Thickness to Urinary Iodine Concentration in Retinitis Pigmentosa With or Without Cystoid Macular Edema. *JAMA Ophthalmology*, *132*(10), 1209-1214. https://doi.org/10.1001/jamaophthalmol.2014.1726
29. Wagner B.D., et al. (2021). Association of Systemic Inflammatory Factors with Progression to Advanced Age-related Macular Degeneration. *Ophthalmic Epidemiology*. https://doi.org/10.1080/09286586.2021.1910314
30. DiNicolantonio, J., & O'Keefe, J. Omega-6 vegetable oils as a driver of coronary heart disease: the oxidized linoleic acid hypothesis. *Open Heart*. *2018*(5), Article e000898. 0.1136/openhrt-2018-000898. https://openheart.bmj.com/content/5/2/e000898
31. Wen, X., et al. (2018). Epigenetics, microbiota, and intraocular inflammation: New paradigms of immune regulation in the eye. *Progress in Retinal and Eye Research*. *64*, 84-95. https://doi.org/10.1016/j.preteyeres.2018.01.001
32. Li, J.J., et al. (2020). Ocular Microbiota and Intraocular Inflammation. *Frontiers in Immunology*, *11*, Article 609765. https://doi.org/10.3389/fimmu.2020.609765
33. Mares J. (2016). Lutein and Zeaxanthin Isomers in Eye Health and Disease. *Annual Review of Nutrition*. *36*, 571–602. https://doi.org/10.1146/annurev-nutr-071715-051110
34. Fassett, R. G., and Coombes, J. S. (2012). Astaxanthin in cardiovascular health and disease. Molecules, *17*(2), 2030–2048. https://doi.org/10.3390/molecules17022030.
35. Dong, Q., et al. (2011). Diversity of bacteria at healthy human conjunctiva. *Investigative Ophthalmology & Visual Science*, *52*(8), 5408–5413. https://doi.org/10.1167/iovs.10-6939
36. Lin C.W., et al. (2020). Protective Effect of Astaxanthin on Blue Light Light-Emitting Diode-Induced Retinal Cell Damage via Free Radical Scavenging and Activation of PI3K/Akt/Nrf2 Pathway in 661W Cell Model. *Marine Drugs*, *18*(8), 387. https://doi.org/10.3390/md18080387
37. Ponce, C., Alfredo, J. (2010). *Phospholipids and Terpenes Enhance the Absorption of Polyphenolics in a CACO-2 Cell Model*. Texas A&M University Office of Graduate Studies. http://oaktrust.library.tamu.edu/bitstream/handle/1969.1/148448/Cardona_Ponce.pdf?sequence=1&isAllowed=y.

NOTES

38. National Eye Institute. (2007, June 24). *Omega-3 Fatty Acids Protect Eyes Against Retinopathy, Study Finds*. National Institutes of Health. https://www.nei.nih.gov/about/news-and-events/news/omega-3-fatty-acids-protect-eyes-against-retinopathy-study-finds
39. Layana, A. G., et al. (2017). Vitamin D and Age-Related Macular Degeneration. *Nutrients*, 9(10), 1120. https://doi.org/10.3390/nu9101120
40. Christen, W.G., et al. (2009). Folic acid, pyridoxine, and cyanocobalamin combination treatment and age-related macular degeneration in women: the Women's Antioxidant and Folic Acid Cardiovascular Study. *Archives of Internal Medicine*, 169(4), 335–341. https://doi.org/10.1001/archinternmed.2008.574

4. MYOPIA & ASTIGMATISM

1. The Eye Diseases Prevalence Research Group. (2004). The Prevalence of Refractive Errors Among Adults in the United States, Western Europe, and Australia. *Archives of Ophthalmology*, 122(4):495–505. https://doi.org/10.1001/archopht.122.4.495
2. Vitale S., et al. (2008). Prevalence of refractive error in the United States, 1999-2004. *Archives of Ophthalmology*, 126(8), 1111-1119. https://doi.org/10.1001/archopht.126.8.1111
3. Holden, B., et al. (2016). Global Prevalence of Myopia and High Myopia and Temporal Trends from 2000 through 2050. *Ophthalmology*, 123(5), 1036-1042. https://www.aaojournal.org/article/S0161-6420(16)00025-7/fulltext
4. Jacewiz, N. (2016, July 7). *What Did Nearsighted Humans Do Before Glasses?* National Public Radio. https://www.npr.org/sections/health-shots/2016/07/07/484835077/what-did-nearsighted-humans-do-before-glasses
5. Heidary, Gena, et al. (2005). The Association of Astigmatism and Spherical Refractive Error in a High Myopia Cohort. *Optometry and Vision Science*, 82(4), 239-243. https://doi.org/10.1097/01.opx.0000159361.17876.96
6. Young, F. A., et al. (1969). The Transmission of Refractive Errors within Eskimo Families. *American Journal of Optometry and*

Archives of the American Academy of Optometry 46(9), 676-685. https://doi.org/10.1097/00006324-196909000-00005

7. Sheedy, J. E., & Shaw-McMinn, P. (2003). *Diagnosing and Treating Computer-Related Vision Problems*. Butterworth-Heinemann. https://doi.org/10.1016/B978-0-7506-7404-1.X5001-1

   ANSES. (2019, May 19). *LEDs: ANSES's recommendations for limiting exposure to blue light*. Republique Francaise. https://www.anses.fr/en/content/leds-anses%E2%80%99s-recommendations-limiting-exposure-blue-light

8. Katz, L., & Berlin, K. (2014). Psychological Stress in Childhood and Myopia Development. *Optometry & Visual Performance*, 2(6), 289-296. https://www.ovpjournal.org/uploads/2/3/8/9/23898265/ovp2-6_article_katz_web.pdf

9. Willis, Jeffrey, et al. (2016). The Prevalence of Myopic Choroidal Neovascularization in the United States. *Ophthalmology*, 123(8), 1771-1782. https://doi.org/10.1016/j.ophtha.2016.04.021

10. Lane, B.C. (1981). *Calcium, Chromium, Protein, Sugar and Accommodation in Myopia*[Conference session]. In Third International Conference on Myopia, Copenhagen, Denmark. https://doi.org/10.1007/978-94-009-8662-6_21

11. Office of Dietary Supplements. (n.d.) *Chromium: Fact Sheet for Health Professionals*. National Institutes of Health. https://ods.od.nih.gov/factsheets/Chromium-HealthProfessional/

12. Crantz, F. *Graves' Disease*. American Thyroid Association. https://www.thyroid.org/patient-thyroid-information/ct-for-patients/vol-7-issue-8/vol-7-issue-8-p-3-4/

13. Ekici, F., et al. The Role of Magnesium in the Pathogenesis and Treatment of Glaucoma. *International Scholarly Research Notices, 2014*, Article 745739. https://www.ncbi.nlm.nih.gov/pmc/articles/PMC4897098/

14. Office of Dietary Supplements. (n.d.). *Omega-3 Fatty Acids: Fact Sheet for Consumers*. National Institutes of Health. https://ods.od.nih.gov/factsheets/Omega3FattyAcids-%20HealthProfessional/

15. Dornstauder, B., et al. (2012). Dietary Docosahexaenoic Acid Supplementation Prevents Age-Related Functional Losses and A2E Accumulation in the Retina. *Investigative Ophthalmology & Visual Science*, 53(4), 2256-2265. https://doi.org/10.1167/iovs.11-8569

NOTES

16. Sreelatha, S., & Inbavalli, R. (2012). Antioxidant, antihyperglycemic, and antihyperlipidemic effects of Coriandrum sativum leaf and stem in alloxan-induced diabetic rats. *Journal of Food and Sciences*, 77(7), T119-T123. https://doi.org/10.1111/j.1750-3841.2012.02755.x
17. Umar A, et al. (2010). Antihypertensive effects of Ocimum basilicum L. (OBL) on blood pressure in renovascular hypertensive rats. *Hypertension Research*, 33, 727-730. https://doi.org/10.1038/hr.2010.64
18. Stoecker, B., et al. (2010). Cinnamon extract lowers blood glucose in hyperglycemic subjects. *The FASEB Journal*, 24(51), 722.1. https://doi.org/10.1096/fasebj.24.1_supplement.722.1
19. Zoladz, P., & Raudenbush, B. (2005). Cognitive Enhancement through Stimulation of the Chemical Senses. *North American Journal of Psychology*, 7, 127. https://www.semanticscholar.org/paper/Cognitive-Enhancement-through-Stimulation-of-the-Zoladz-Raudenbush/99077e8eb8ffb81a041488721f3985f68d09b1f5#paper-header
20. Singh, G., et al. (2007). A comparison of chemical, antioxidant and antimicrobial studies of cinnamon leaf and bark volatile oils, oleoresins and their constituents. *Food and Chemical Toxicology*, 45, 1650-1661. https://www.cinnamonvogue.com/DOWNLOADS/antioxidant-and-antimicrobial-studies-of-cinnamon-leaf-and-bark-volatile-oils-oleoresins1.pdf
21. Harvard Health Publishing. (2010, October 12). *A prescription for better health: Go alfresco*. https://www.health.harvard.edu/mind-and-mood/a-prescription-for-better-health-go-alfresco
22. Louv, R. (2019, October) *What is Nature-Deficit Disorder?* Children and Nature Network. https://www.childrenandnature.org/resources/what-is-nature-deficit-disorder/
23. Rose, K.A., et al. (2008). Outdoor activity reduces the prevalence of myopia in children. *Ophthalmology*, 115(8), 1279-1285. https://doi.org/10.1016/j.ophtha.2007.12.019
24. American Optometric Association. (n.d.). *Computer vision syndrome*. https://www.aoa.org/healthy-eyes/eye-and-vision-conditions/computer-vision-syndrome?sso=y.

NOTES

5. HYPEROPIA & PRESBYOPIA

1. National Eye Institute. (2019, July 17). *Farsightedness (Hyperopia) Data and Statistics*. https://www.nei.nih.gov/learn-about-eye-health/outreach-campaigns-and-resources/eye-health-data-and-statistics/farsightedness-hyperopia-data-and-statistics.
2. Grigorian, P. (2015, January 6). *Eyewiki: Hyperopia*. American Academy of Ophthalmology. https://eyewiki.aao.org/Hyperopia#cite_ref-paispe_14-0
3. Patel, I. et al. (2007) Presbyopia: prevalence, impact, and interventions. *Community Eye Health, 20*(63), 40-41. https://www.ncbi.nlm.nih.gov/pmc/articles/PMC2040246/
4. Borchert, M.S., et al. (2011). Multi-Ethnic Pediatric Eye Disease Study and the Baltimore Pediatric Eye Disease Study Groups. Risk factors for hyperopia and myopia in preschool children: The multi-ethnic pediatric eye disease and Baltimore pediatric eye disease studies. *Ophthalmology, 118*(10), 1966-1973. https://doi.org/10.1016/j.ophtha.2011.06.030
5. Padhye, A.S., et al. (2009). Prevalence of uncorrected refractive error and other eye problems among urban and rural school children. *Middle East African Journal of Ophthalmology, 16*(2), 69-74. http://www.meajo.org/article.asp?issn=0974-9233;year=2009;volume=16;issue=2;spage=69;epage=74;aulast=Padhye
6. Genetics Home Reference. (n.d.). *Farsightedness*. MedlinePlus. https://medlineplus.gov/genetics/condition/farsightedness/
7. Mayo Clinic Staff. (n.d.). *Presbyopia*. Mayo Clinic. https://www.mayoclinic.org/diseases-conditions/presbyopia/symptoms-causes/syc-20363328
8. Grigorian, P. (2015, January 6). *Eyewiki: Hyperopia*. American Academy of Ophthalmology. https://eyewiki.aao.org/Hyperopia#cite_ref-paispe_14-0
9. Williams W.R., et al. (2005). Hyperopia and educational attainment in a primary school cohort. *Archives of Disease in Childhood, 2005*(90), 150-153. http://dx.doi.org/10.1136/adc.2003.046755
10. Moon B.Y., et al. (2019). Effect of induced hyperopia on fall risk and Fourier transformation of postural sway. *PeerJ, 7*, Article e8329. https://doi.org/10.7717/peerj.8329

NOTES

11. Askari, G., et al. (2012). The effect of quercetin supplementation on selected markers of inflammation and oxidative stress. *Journal of research in medical sciences, 17*(7), 637–641. https://www.ncbi.nlm.nih.gov/pmc/articles/PMC3685779/
12. Armenta, A. (2021). *Presbyopia Surgery.* Vision Center. https://www.visioncenter.org/refractive-errors/presbyopia/surgery/.
13. Ibid.
14. Mukamal, R. (2021, March 24). *Corneal Inlays: A Surgical Alternative to Reading Glasses.* American Academy of Ophthalmology. https://www.aao.org/eye-health/treatments/corneal-inlays-alternative-to-reading-glasses
15. Boyd, K. (2018, May 7). *What Is Monovision (or Blended Vision)?.* American Academy of Ophthalmology. https://www.aao.org/eye-health/treatments/what-is-monovision-blended-vision

6. STRABISMUS, AMBLYOPIA, AND DIPLOPIA

1. Centers for Disease Control and Prevention. (n.d.). *Common Eye Disorders and Diseases.* https://www.cdc.gov/visionhealth/basics/ced/index.html.
2. Ibid.
3. National Eye Institute. (2019, July 2). *Amblyopia (Lazy Eye).* https://www.nei.nih.gov/learn-about-eye-health/eye-conditions-and-diseases/amblyopia-lazy-eye
4. Cleveland Clinic. (n.d.). *Strabismus (Crossed Eyes).* https://my.clevelandclinic.org/health/diseases/15065-strabismus-crossed-eyes
5. Mayo Clinic. *Lazy eye (amblyopia).* https://www.mayoclinic.org/diseases-conditions/lazy-eye/symptoms-causes/syc-20352391#:~:text=Lazy%20eye%20(amblyopia)%20is%20reduced,lazy%20eye%20affects%20both%20eyes
6. Simborg, M.. (2017, March 4). *Lazy Eye Surgery Facts.* American Academy of Ophthalmology. https://www.aao.org/eye-health/tips-prevention/lazy-eye-surgery-facts
7. Review of Optometry. (2009, July 1) *An Interview with 'Stereo Sue'.* https://www.reviewofoptometry.com/article/an-interview-with-stereo-sue

NOTES

8. Dennis S.C., et al. (2011). Adjunctive Effect of Acupuncture to Refractive Correction on Anisometropic Amblyopia: One Year Results of a Randomized Crossover Trial. *Ophthalmology, 118*(8), 1501-1511. https://doi.org/10.1016/j.ophtha.2011.01.017
9. Zhao, J., et al. (2010). Randomized controlled trial of patching vs acupuncture for anisometropic amblyopia in children aged 7 to 12 years. *JAMA Ophthalmology, 128*(12), 1510-1517. https://doi.org/10.1001/archophthalmol.2010.306
10. Do, A., et al. (2014). Acupuncture treatment of diplopia associated with abducens palsy: a case report. *Global Advances in Health and Medicine, 3*(4), 32-34. https://doi.org/10.7453/gahmj.2014.024
11. Quraishy, K. (2016). Feeding in the NICU: A Perspective from a Craniosacral Therapist. *Neonatal Network, 35*(2), 105-7. https://doi.org/10.1891/0730-0832.35.2.105
12. Buscemi, S., et al. (2018). The Effect of Lutein on Eye and Extra-Eye Health. *Nutrients, 10*(9), 1321. https://doi.org/10.3390/nu10091321
13. Mykkänen, O. T., et al. (2012). Bilberries potentially alleviate stress-related retinal gene expression induced by a high-fat diet in mice. *Molecular Vision. 18*, 2338–2351. https://www.ncbi.nlm.nih.gov/pmc/articles/PMC3444297/.
14. Ozawa, Y., et al. (2015). Bilberry extract supplementation for preventing eye fatigue in video display terminal workers. *The Journal of Nutrition, Health, and Aging, 19*, 548-554. https://doi.org/10.1007/s12603-014-0573-6
15. Froger, N., et al. (2012). Taurine provides neuroprotection against retinal ganglion cell degeneration. *PLoS One. 7*(10), Article e42017. https://doi.org/10.1371/journal.pone.0042017. https://journals.plos.org/plosone/article?id=10.1371/journal.pone.0042017
16. Militante, J.D., & Lombardini, J.B. (2002). Taurine: evidence of physiological function in the retina. *Nutritional Neuroscience, 5*(2), 75-90. https://doi.org/10.1080/10284150290018991
17. Review of Optometry. (2009, July 1) *An Interview with Stereo Sue.* https://www.reviewofoptometry.com/article/an-interview-with-stereo-sue.

NOTES

7. DRUGS AND SURGERY VERSUS HERBS AND AROMATHERAPY

1. Miller, D., and Iovieno, A. (2009) The role of microbial flora on the ocular surface. *Current Opinion in Allergy and Clinical Immunology*, 9(5), 466-470. https://doi.org/10.1097/ACI.0b013e3283303e1b
2. Keiltey, R. (1930). The Bacterial Flora of the Normal Conjunctive with Comparative Nasal Culture Study. *American Journal of Ophthalmology*, 13(10), 876-879. https://doi.org/10.1016/S0002-9394(30)92437-3.
3. Doan, T., et al. (2016)."Paucibacterial Microbiome and Resident DNA Virome of the Healthy Conjunctiva. *Investigative Ophthalmology & Visual Science*, 57(13), 5116-5126. https://doi.org/10.1167/iovs.16-19803
4. Li, Z.Y., et al. (1985). Amelioration of photic injury in rat retina by ascorbic acid: a histopathologic study. *Investigative Ophthalmology & Visual Science*, 26(11), 1589-98. https://iovs.arvojournals.org/article.aspx?articleid=2159645
5. Lee, S.H., et al. (2012). Comparative ocular microbial communities in humans with and without blepharitis. *Investigative Ophthalmology & Visual Science*, 53(9), 5585-5593. https://doi.org/10.1167/iovs.12-9922
6. Berry, M., et al. (2002). Commensal ocular bacteria degrade mucins. *The British Journal of Ophthalmology*, 86, 1412–1416. https://doi.org/10.1136/bjo.86.12.1412
7. Graham, J.E., et al. (2007). Ocular pathogen or commensal: a PCR-based study of surface bacterial flora in normal and dry eyes. *Investigative Ophthalmology & Visual Science*, 48(12), 5616-5623. https://doi.org/10.1167/iovs.07-0588
8. Andriessen, E. M., et al. (2016). Gut microbiota influences pathological angiogenesis in obesity-driven choroidal neovascularization. *EMBO Molecular Medicine*, 8(12), 1366–1379. https://doi.org/10.15252/emmm.201606531
9. Levine, J. S., & Burakoff, R. (2011). Extraintestinal manifestations of inflammatory bowel disease. *Gastroenterology & Hepatology*, 7(4), 235–241. https://www.ncbi.nlm.nih.gov/pmc/articles/PMC3127025/

10. Zarate-Blades, C. R., et al. (2017). Gut microbiota as a source of a surrogate antigen that triggers autoimmunity in an immune privileged site. *Gut Microbes, 8*,(1), 59-66. http://dx.doi.org/10.1080/19490976.2016.1273996

11. Berry, M., et al. (2002). Commensal ocular bacteria degrade mucins. *The British Journal of Ophthalmology, 86*(12), 1412–1416. https://doi.org/10.1136/bjo.86.12.1412

12. Shin, H., et al. (2016). Changes in the Eye Microbiota Associated with Contact Lens Wearing. mBio, 7(2), Article e00198. https://doi.org/10.1128/mBio.00198-16

13. Centers for Disease Control and Prevention. (n.d.). *Antibiotic Resistance Questions and Answers.* https://www.cdc.gov/antibiotic-use/antibiotic-resistance.html?CDC_AA_refVal=https%3A%2F%2Fwww.cdc.gov%2Fantibiotic-use%2Fcommunity%2Fabout%2Fantibiotic-resistance-faqs.html

14. Review on Antimicrobial Resistance. (2014). *Review on Antimicrobial Resistance. Antimicrobial Resistance: Tackling a Crisis for the Health and Wealth of Nations.* https://amr-review.org/sites/default/files/AMR%20Review%20Paper%20-%20Tackling%20a%20crisis%20for%20the%20health%20and%20wealth%20of%20nations_1.pdf

15. Kresser, C. (2018, July 10) *The Ocular Microbiome, with Dr. Harvey Fishman.* ChrisKresser. https://chriskresser.com/the-ocular-microbiome-with-dr-harvey-fishman/.

16. Eguchi, H., et al. (2018). Investigation of the perioperative disturbances in the ocular surface microbiome using next-generation sequencing analysis. *Investigative Ophthalmology & Visual Science, 59*(9), 3688. https://iovs.arvojournals.org/article.aspx?articleid=2691492

17. Vetter, M. L. & Hitchcock, P., F.. Report on the National Eye Institute Audacious Goals Initiative: Replacement of Retinal Ganglion Cells from Endogenous Cell Sources. *Translational Vision Science & Technology* 6(2), 5. https://doi.org/10.1167/tvst.6.2.5

18. Jorstad, N.L., et al. (2017). Stimulation of functional neuronal regeneration from Müller glia in adult mice. *Nature, 548*, 103-107. https://doi.org/10.1038/nature23283

19. Zhang, J., et al. (2016). The Neuroprotective Properties of Hericium erinaceus in Glutamate-Damaged Differentiated PC12 Cells and an Alzheimer's Disease Mouse Model. *International Journal of*

NOTES

Molecular Sciences, 17(11), 1810. https://doi.org/10.3390/ijms17111810

20. Weber, A. J., et al. (2010). Combined application of BDNF to the eye and brain enhances ganglion cell survival and function in the cat after optic nerve injury. *Investigative Ophthalmology & Visual Science, 51*(1), 327–334. https://doi.org/10.1167/iovs.09-3740

21. Weinstein, G., et al. (2014). Serum Brain-Derived Neurotrophic Factor and the Risk for Dementia: The Framingham Heart Study. *JAMA Neurology, 71*(1), 55-61. https://jamanetwork.com/journals/jamaneurology/fullarticle/1779513

22. Sarraf, P., et Al. (2019). Short-term curcumin supplementation enhances serum brain-derived neurotrophic factor in adult men and women: a systematic review and dose=response meta-analysis of randomized controlled trials. *Nutrition Research, 69*, 1-8. https://www.sciencedirect.com/science/article/pii/S0271531719301009

23. Travaglia, A., & La Mendola, D. (2017). Zinc Interactions With Brain-Derived Neurotrophic Factor and Related Peptide Fragments. *Vitamins and Hormones, 104*, 29-56. https://pubmed.ncbi.nlm.nih.gov/28215299/

24. Lee, H.J., et al. (2019). Sodium butyrate prevents radiation-induced cognitive impairment by restoring pCREB/BDNF expression. *Neural Regeneration Research. 14*(9), 1530–1535. https://doi.org/10.4103/1673-5374.255974

25. Iovieno, A. (2006). Probiotic Eye–Drops Treatment in Patients Affected by Vernal Keratoconjunctivitis. *Investigative Ophthalmology and Visual Science, 47*(13), 4998. https://iovs.arvojournals.org/article.aspx?articleid=2394783

26. Boire, N., et al. (2013). Essential Oils and Future Antibiotics: New Weapons against Emerging 'Superbugs'? *Journal of Infectious Diseases and Preventive Medicine, 1*(2), Article 1000105. https://www.longdom.org/open-access/essential-oils-and-future-antibiotics-new-weapons-against-emerging-superbugs-2329-8731.1000105.pdf

27. de Rapper, S., et al. (2012). The additive and synergistic antimicrobial effects of select frankincense and myrrh oils--a combination from the pharaonic pharmacopoeia. *Letters in Applied Microbiology, 54*(4), 352-8. https://doi.org/10.1111/j.1472-765X.2012.03216.x

NOTES

28. al-Hader, A.A., et al. (1994). Hyperglycemic and insulin release inhibitory effects of Rosmarinus officinalis. *Journal of Ethnopharmacology, 43*(3), 217-21. https://pubmed.ncbi.nlm.nih.gov/7990497/
29. Chung, M.J., et al. (2010). Anti-diabetic effects of lemon balm (Melissa officinalis) essential oil on glucose- and lipid-regulating enzymes in type 2 diabetic mice. *British Journal of Nutrition, 104*(2),180-188. https://doi.org/10.1017/S0007114510001765
30. Hajhashemi, V., et al. (2003). Anti-inflammatory and analgesic properties of the leaf extracts and essential oil of Lavandula angustifolia Mill. *Journal of Ethnopharmacology, 89*(1), 67-71. https://pubmed.ncbi.nlm.nih.gov/14522434/
31. Bellassoued, K., et al. (2018). Protective effects of Mentha piperita L. leaf essential oil against CCl4 induced hepatic oxidative damage and renal failure in rats. *Lipids in Health and Disease, 17*(9), 1-14. https://www.ncbi.nlm.nih.gov/pmc/articles/PMC5761127/
32. Al-Shuneigat, J., et al. Effects of a topical essential oil-containing formulation on biofilm-forming coagulase-negative staphylococci. *Letters in Applied Microbiology. 41*, 52-55. https://doi.org/10.1111/j.1472-765X.2005.01699.x
33. Schuhmacher, A., et al. (2003). Virucidal effect of peppermint oil on the enveloped viruses herpes simplex virus type 1 and type 2 in vitro. *Phytomedicine, 10*(6-7), 504-10. https://doi.org/10.1078/094471103322331467
34. Benencia, F. & Courreges, M.C. (1999). Antiviral activity of sandalwood oil against Herpes simplex viruses-1 and -2. *Phytomedicine, 6*(2), 119-123. https://pubmed.ncbi.nlm.nih.gov/10374251/
35. Garozzo, A., et al. (2011). Activity of Melaleuca alternifolia (tea tree) oil on Influenza virus A/PR/8: study on the mechanism of action. *Antiviral Research, 89*(1), 83-8. https://doi.org/10.1016/j.antiviral.2010.11.010
36. Brady, A., et al. (2006). In vitro activity of tea-tree oil against clinical skin isolates of meticillin-resistant and -sensitive staphylococcus aureus and coagulase-negative staphylococci growing planktonically and as biofilms. *Journal of Medical Microbiology* (Pt 10), 1375-1380.

NOTES

37. Burt, S.A., and Reinders, R.D. (2003). Antibacterial activity of selected plant essential oils against Escherichia coli O157:H7. *Letters in Applied Microbiology*, 36(3):162-167. https://doi.org/10.1046/j.1472-765x.2003.01285.x
38. Hammer, K.A., et al. (2004). Antifungal effects of Melaleuca alternifolia (tea tree) oil and its components on Candida albicans, Candida glabrata and Saccharomyces cerevisiae. *Journal of Antimicrobial Chemotherapy*, 53(6), 1081-5. https://doi.org/10.1093/jac/dkh243
39. Pina-Vaz, C., et al. (2004). Antifungal activity of Thymus oils and their major compounds. *Journal of the European Academy of Dermatology and Venereology*, 18(1), 73-78. https://doi.org/10.1111/j.1468-3083.2004.00886.x
40. Cappello, G., et al. (2007). Peppermint oil (Mintoil) in the treatment of irritable bowel syndrome: a prospective double blind placebo-controlled randomized trial. *Digestive and liver disease : official journal of the Italian Society of Gastroenterology and the Italian Association for the Study of the Liver*, 39(6), 530-536. https://doi.org/10.1016/j.dld.2007.02.006
41. Anderson, L.A., and Gross JB. (2004). Aromatherapy with peppermint, isopropyl alcohol, or placebo is equally effective in relieving postoperative nausea. *Journal of Perianesthesia Nursing*, 19(1), 29-35. https://doi.org/10.1016/j.jopan.2003.11.001
42. Alexandrovich I, et al. (2003). The effect of fennel (Foeniculum Vulgare) seed oil emulsion in infantile colic: a randomized, placebo-controlled study. *Alternative Therapies in Health and Medicine*, 9(4), 58-61. https://pubmed.ncbi.nlm.nih.gov/12868253/

8. NUTRITION TIPS – WHAT TO EAT FOR HEALTHY EYES

1. Chiu, C.H., et al. (2018). Erinacine A-Enriched Hericium erinaceus Mycelium Produces Antidepressant-Like Effects through Modulating BDNF/PI3K/Akt/GSK-3β Signaling in Mice. *International Journal of Molecular Sciences*, 19(2), 341. https://doi.org/10.3390/ijms19020341
2. Fowler, S. P., et al. (2015). Diet soda intake is associated with long-term increases in waist circumference in a biethnic cohort of

older adults: the San Antonio Longitudinal Study of Aging. *Journal of the American Geriatrics Society*, 63(4), 708–715. https://doi.org/10.1111/jgs.13376.

3. Sanda, B. (2004, February 19). *The Double Danger of High Fructose Corn Syrup*. The Weston A. Price Foundation. westonaprice.org/health-topics/modern-foods/the-double-danger-of-high-fructose-corn-syrup/.

4. Dufault, R., et al. (2009). Mercury from chlor-alkali plants: measured concentrations in food product sugar. *Environmental Health*, 8, Article 2. https://ehjournal.biomedcentral.com/articles/10.1186/1476-069X-8-2.

5. Liu, H., et al. (2010). Fructose Induces Transketolase Flux to Promote Pancreatic Cancer Growth. *Cancer Research*, 70(15), 6368-6376. https://doi.org/10.1158/0008-5472.CAN-09-4615

6. Harvard Health Publishing. (2011, September 1). *Abundance of fructose not good for the liver, heart*. https://www.health.harvard.edu/heart-health/abundance-of-fructose-not-good-for-the-liver-heart

7. National Cancer Institute. (2018, December 28). *Aflatoxins*. https://www.cancer.gov/about-cancer/causes-prevention/risk/substances/aflatoxins.

8. Gershon, M. (1999). *The Second Brain: A Groundbreaking New Understanding of Nervous Disorders of the Stomach and Intestine*. Harper Perennial.

9. Lassale, C., et al. (2019). Healthy dietary indices and risk of depressive outcomes: a systematic review and meta-analysis of observational studies. *Molecular Psychiatry*, 24(7), 965–986. https://doi.org/10.1038/s41380-018-0237-8

10. LaChance, L. R., & Ramsey, D. (2018). Antidepressant foods: An evidence-based nutrient profiling system for depression. *World Journal of Psychiatry*, 8(3), 97–104. https://doi.org/10.5498/wjp.v8.i3.97

11. Clapp, M., et al. (2017). Gut microbiota's effect on mental health: The gut-brain axis. *Clinics and Practice*, 7(4), 131-136. https://doi.org/10.4081/cp.2017.987

12. Qiao, Y., et al. (2013). Alterations of the gut microbiota in high-fat diet mice is strongly linked to oxidative stress. *Applied Microbiology & Biotechnology*, 97(4), 1689-97. https://doi.org/10.1007/s00253-012-4323-6

NOTES

13. Pierre, J. F., et al. (2018). Dietary antioxidant micronutrients alter mucosal inflammatory risk in a murine model of genetic and microbial susceptibility. *The Journal of Nutritional Biochemistry, 54*, 95–104. https://doi.org/10.1016/j.jnutbio.2017.12.002
14. National Institute of Health: National Center for Complementary and Integrative Health. (2013, November). *Antioxidants: In Depth.* https://www.nccih.nih.gov/health/antioxidants-in-depth
15. Imran, M., et al. (2020). Lycopene as a Natural Antioxidant Used to Prevent Human Health Disorders. *Antioxidants, 9*(8), 706. https://doi.org/10.3390/antiox9080706
16. Rowles, J. L. III, et al. (2017). Increased dietary and circulating lycopene are associated with reduced prostate cancer risk: a systematic review and meta-analysis. *Prostate Cancer and Prostatic Diseases, 20*(4), 361-377. https://doi.org/10.1038/pcan.2017.25
17. Rowles, J.L. III, et al. (2018). Processed and raw tomato consumption and risk of prostate cancer: a systematic review and dose-response meta-analysis. *Prostate Cancer and Prostatic Diseases, 21*(3), 319-336. https://doi.org/10.1038/s41391-017-0005-x
18. Mozos, I., et al. (2018). Lycopene and Vascular Health. *Frontiers in pharmacology, 9*, 521. https://doi.org/10.3389/fphar.2018.00521
19. Chen D, et al. (2019). A review for the pharmacological effect of lycopene in central nervous system disorders. *Biomedicine & Pharmacotherapy, 111*, 791-801. https://www.sciencedirect.com/science/article/pii/S0753332218374869?via%3Dihub
20. Radmehr, M., et al. (2016). Comparison of the Effect of Lycopene with Ibuprofen on Sensory Threshold of Pain Using Formalin Test in Adult Male Rats. *Journal of Chemical and Pharmaceutical Research, 8*(4),1322-1327. https://www.jocpr.com/articles/comparison-of-the-effect-of-lycopene-with-ibuprofen-on-sensory-threshold-of-pain-using-formalin-test-in-adult-male-rats.pdf
21. Jenkins, G., et al. (2014). Wrinkle reduction in post-menopausal women consuming a novel oral supplement: a double-blind placebo-controlled randomized study. *International Journal of Cosmetic Science, 36*(1), 22-31. https://doi.org/10.1111/ics.12087
22. Stahl, W., et al. (2001). Dietary Tomato Paste Protects Against Ultraviolet Light-induced Erythema in Humans. *The Journal of Nutrition, 131*(5), 1449-1451. https://academic.oup.com/jn/article/131/5/1449/4686953

23. Grether-Beck, S., et al. (2017). Molecular evidence that oral supplementation with lycopene or lutein protects human skin against ultraviolet radiation: results from a double-blinded, placebo-controlled, crossover study. *British Journal of Dermatology, 176*, 1120-1121. https://onlinelibrary.wiley.com/doi/epdf/10.1111/bjd.15080
24. Tan, B. L., & Norhaizan, M. E. (2019). Carotenoids: How Effective Are They to Prevent Age-Related Diseases?. *Molecules, 24*(9), 1801. https://doi.org/10.3390/molecules24091801
25. Johnson, E.J. (2002). The Role of Carotenoids in Human Health. *Nutrition in Clinical Care, 5*(2), 56-65. https://doi.org/10.1046/j.1523-5408.2002.00004.x
26. Grodstein, F., et al. (2007). A randomized trial of beta carotene supplementation and cognitive function in men: the Physicians' Health Study II. *Archives of Internal Medicine, 167*(20), 2184-90. https://doi.org/10.1001/archinte.167.20.2184
27. Hu, P., et al. (2006). Association between serum beta-carotene levels and decline of cognitive function in high-functioning older persons with or without apolipoprotein E 4 alleles: MacArthur studies of successful aging. *The Journals of Gerontology: Series A Biological Sciences and Medical Sciences, 61*(6), 616-20. https://doi.org/10.1093/gerona/61.6.616
28. Beth Israel Lahey Health Winchester Hospital. (n.d.). *Citrus Bioflavonoids.* https://www.winchesterhospital.org/health-library/article?id=21574
29. Homayouni, F., et al. (2018). Blood pressure lowering and anti-inflammatory effects of hesperidin in type 2 diabetes; a randomized double-blind controlled clinical trial. *Phytotherapy Research, 32*(6), 1073-1079. https://doi.org/10.1002/ptr.6046
30. Forte, R., et al. (2013). Long-term follow-up of oral administration of flavonoids, Centella asiatica and Melilotus, for diabetic cystoid macular edema without macular thickening. *Journal of Ocular Pharmacology and Therapeutics, 29*(8), 733-737. https://doi.org/10.1089/jop.2013.0010
31. Wagner, B.D., et al. (2021). Association of Systemic Inflammatory Factors with Progression to Advanced Age-related Macular Degeneration. *Ophthalmic Epidemiology*, 1-10. https://doi.org/10.1080/09286586.2021.1910314

NOTES

32. Eisenhauer, B., et al. (2017). Lutein and Zeaxanthin-Food Sources, Bioavailability and Dietary Variety in Age-Related Macular Degeneration Protection. *Nutrients, 9*(2), 120. https://doi.org/10.3390/nu9020120

33. Bose, C., et al. (2018). Sulforaphane potentiates anticancer effects of doxorubicin and attenuates its cardiotoxicity in a breast cancer model. *PloS One, 13*(3), Article e0193918. https://doi.org/10.1371/journal.pone.0193918.

34. Kensler, T.W., et al. (2005). Effects of glucosinolate-rich broccoli sprouts on urinary levels of aflatoxin-DNA adducts and phenanthrene tetraols in a randomized clinical trial in He Zuo township, Qidong, People's Republic of China. *Cancer Epidemiology: Biomarkers and Prevention. 14*(11), 2605-2613. https://doi.org/10.1158/1055-9965.EPI-05-0368

35. Kikuchi, M., et al. (2015). Sulforaphane-rich broccoli sprout extract improves hepatic abnormalities in male subjects. *World Journal of Gastroenterology, 21*(43), 12457–12467. https://doi.org/10.3748/wjg.v21.i43.12457.

36. Kong, L., et al. (2016). The therapeutic potential of sulforaphane on light-induced photoreceptor degeneration through antiapoptosis and antioxidant protection. *Neurochemistry International, 100*, 52-61. https://doi.org/10.1016/j.neuint.2016.08.011

37. Blesso, C. N. (2019). Dietary Anthocyanins and Human Health. *Nutrients, 11*(9), 2107. https://doi.org/10.3390/nu11092107

38. Khoo, H. E., et al. (2017). Anthocyanidins and anthocyanins: colored pigments as food, pharmaceutical ingredients, and the potential health benefits. *Food & Nutrition Research, 61*, Article 1361779. https://doi.org/10.1080/16546628.2017.1361779

39. Nomi, Y., et al. (2019). Therapeutic Effects of Anthocyanins for Vision and Eye Health. *Molecules, 24*(18), 3311. https://doi.org/10.3390/molecules24183311

40. Aliahmadi, Mitra, et al. (2021). Effects of raw red beetroot consumption on metabolic markers and cognitive function in type 2 diabetes patients. *Journal of Diabetes & Metabolic Disorders, 20*, 673-682. https://link.springer.com/article/10.1007/s40200-021-00798-z

41. Rahimi, P., et al. (2019). Betalains, the nature-inspired pigments, in health and diseases." *Critical Reviews in Food, Science and Nutri-*

tion, *59*(18), 2949-2978. https://doi.org/10.1080/10408398.2018.1479830

42. Li, Y., et al. (2016). Quercetin, Inflammation and Immunity. *Nutrients, 8*(3), 167. https://doi.org/10.3390/nu8030167

43. Turati, F., et al. (2015). Allium vegetable intake and gastric cancer: a case-control study and meta-analysis. *Molecular Nutrition and Food Research, 59*(1), 171-179. https://doi.org/10.1002/mnfr.201400496

44. Dhawan V, and Jain S. (2005). Garlic supplementation prevents oxidative DNA damage in essential hypertension. *Molecular and Cellular Biochemistry, 275*(1-2), 85-94. https://doi.org/10.1007/s11010-005-0824-2

45. Ashraf, R., et al. (2013). Effects of Allium sativum (garlic) on systolic and diastolic blood pressure in patients with essential hypertension. *Pakistan Journal of Pharmaceutical Sciences.*, *26*(5), 859-63. https://pubmed.ncbi.nlm.nih.gov/24035939/

46. Kianoush, S., et al. (2012). Comparison of therapeutic effects of garlic and d-Penicillamine in patients with chronic occupational lead poisoning. *Basic and Clinical Pharmacology and Toxicology, 110*(5), 476-81. https://doi.org/10.1111/j.1742-7843.2011.00841.x

47. Bayan, L., et al. (2014). Garlic: a review of potential therapeutic effects. *Avicenna Journal of Phytomedicine, 4*(1), 1–14. https://www.ncbi.nlm.nih.gov/pmc/articles/PMC4103721/

48. Zhang, J. J., et al. (2016). Bioactivities and Health Benefits of Mushrooms Mainly from China. *Molecules, 21*(7), 938. https://doi.org/10.3390/molecules21070938.

49. Blagodatski, A., et al. (2018). Medicinal mushrooms as an attractive new source of natural compounds for future cancer therapy. *Oncotarget, 9*(49), 29259–29274. https://doi.org/10.18632/oncotarget.25660

50. Brown, M.J., et al. (2004). Carotenoid bioavailability is higher from salads ingested with full-fat than with fat-reduced salad dressings as measured with electrochemical detection. *American Journal of Clinical Nutrition, 80*(2), 396-403. https://doi.org/10.1093/ajcn/80.2.396

51. Shmerling, R. (2017, September 25). *The latest scoop on the health benefits of coffee.* Harvard Health Blog. https://www.health.harvard.edu/blog/the-latest-scoop-on-the-health-benefits-of-coffee-2017092512429

NOTES

52. Yokosawa, T., & Dong, E. (1997). Influence of green tea and its three major components upon low-density lipoprotein oxidation. *Pathology*, 49(5), 329-335. https://www.sciencedirect.com/science/article/pii/S0940299397800966

53. Hartley, L., et al. (2013). *Green and black tea for the primary prevention of cardiovascular disease.* Cochrane Database of Systematic Reviews. https://www.cochranelibrary.com/cdsr/doi/10.1002/14651858.CD009934.pub2/full

54. Eng, Q.Y., et al. (2018). Molecular understanding of Epigallocatechin gallate (EGCG) in cardiovascular and metabolic diseases. *Journal of Ethnopharmacology*, 210, 296-310. https://doi.org/10.1016/j.jep.2017.08.035

55. Weinreb, O., et al. (2004). Neurological mechanisms of green tea polyphenols in Alzheimer's and Parkinson's diseases. *Journal of Nutritional Biochemistry*, 15(9), 506-16. https://doi.org/10.1016/j.jnutbio.2004.05.002

56. Nathan PJ, et al. (2006). The neuropharmacology of L-theanine(N-ethyl-L-glutamine): a possible neuroprotective and cognitive enhancing agent. *Journal of Herbal Pharmacotherapy*, 6(2), 21-30. https://pubmed.ncbi.nlm.nih.gov/17182482/

57. Liu, K., et al. (2013). Effect of green tea on glucose control and insulin sensitivity: a meta-analysis of 17 randomized controlled trials. *The American Journal of Clinical Nutrition*, 98(2), 340-348. https://academic.oup.com/ajcn/article/98/2/340/4577179

58. Iso, H., et al. (2006). The relationship between green tea and total caffeine intake and risk for self-reported type 2 diabetes among Japanese adults. *Annals of International Medicine*, 144(8), 554-62. https://doi.org/10.7326/0003-4819-144-8-200604180-00005

59. Laitano, O., et al. (2014). Improved exercise capacity in the heat followed by coconut water consumption, *Motriz, Rio Claro*, 20(1), 107-111. http://dx.doi.org/10.1590/S1980-65742014000100016.

60. Geetha, V., et al. (2016). Effect of Shelf Stable Concentrates of Tender Coconut Water and Testa Phenolics on Lipid Profile and Liver Antioxidant Enzymes in High Fat Fed Rats. *Global Journal of Biology, Agriculture & Health Sciences*, 5(2), 25-30. https://www.longdom.org/articles/effect-of-shelf-stable-concentrates-of-tender-coconut-water-and-testa-phenolics-on-lipid-profile-and-liver-antioxidant-e.pdf

61. Preetha, P.P., et al. (2015). Mature coconut water exhibits antidiabetic and antithrombotic potential via L-arginine-nitric oxide pathway in alloxan induced diabetic rats. *Journal of Basic and Clinical Physiology and Pharmacology*, 26(6), 575-83. https://doi.org/10.1515/jbcpp-2014-0126
62. Kalt, W., et al. (2014). Blueberry effects on dark vision and recovery after photobleaching: placebo-controlled crossover studies. *Journal of Agricultural and Food Chemistry.*, 62(46), 11180-9. https://doi.org/10.1021/jf503689c
63. Song, Y., et al. (2016). Effects of blueberry anthocyanins on retinal oxidative stress and inflammation in diabetes through Nrf2/HO-1 signaling. *Journal of Neuroimmunology*. 301, 1-6. https://doi.org/10.1016/j.jneuroim.2016.11.001
64. Intahphuak, S., et al. (2010). Anti-inflammatory, analgesic, and antipyretic activities of virgin coconut oil. *Pharmaceutical Biology*, 48(2), 151-157. https://doi.org/10.3109/13880200903062614
65. Nafar, F., et al. (2017). Coconut oil protects cortical neurons from amyloid beta toxicity by enhancing signaling of cell survival pathways. *Neurochemistry International*, 105, 64-79. https://doi.org/10.1016/j.neuint.2017.01.008
66. Lerdweeraphon, W., et al. (2013). Perinatal taurine exposure affects adult oxidative stress. *American Journal of Physiology: Regulatory Integrative and Comparative Physiology*, , 305(2), R95-R97. https://doi.org/10.1152/ajpregu.00142.2013

9. LIGHT, COLOR, AND VIBRATIONAL MEDICINE FOR HEALING THE EYES AND BODY

1. Wolken, J.J. (1961). The Photoreceptor Structures. *International Review of Cytology*, 1961. 11, 195-218.
2. Brainard, G., et al. (2001). Action Spectrum for Melatonin Regulation in Humans; Evidence for a Novel Circadian Photoreceptor. *Journal of Neuroscience*, 21(16), 6405-6412. https://doi.org/10.1523/JNEUROSCI.21-16-06405.2001
3. Slominski, A. T., et al. (2018). How UV Light Touches the Brain and Endocrine System Through Skin, and Why. *Endocrinology*,

NOTES

159(5), https://doi.org/10.1210/en.2017-03230

4. Rojas, J. C., and Gonzalez-Lima, F. (2011). Low-level light therapy of the eye and brain. *Eye and Brain, 3,* 49–67. https://doi.org/10.2147/EB.S21391
5. Ott, John. (1973). *Health and Light*. Reprint - Pocket Books. New York. 2000. (original 1973).
6. Patel, D., et al. (2020, September). *Ocushield: Blue light. How does it affect us?.* Ocushield/AzulOptics. https://cdn.shopify.com/s/files/1/0456/7983/7343/files/How_does_blue_light_affect_us_-_White_paper_clinician_version.pdf?v=1606417042.
7. Lawwill, T. (1975). Mechanisms of retinal damage from chronic laser radiation, thresholds and mechanisms. Report no. 4 (annual) 1 November 1976-31 October 1977. https://www.semanticscholar.org/paper/Mechanisms-of-retinal-damage-from-chronic-laser-and-Lawwill-Crockett/8cd4b6cf672186a646460adf03411a83fe1559c2
8. Ham, W.T., et al. (1976). Retinal sensitivity to damage from short wavelength light. *Nature, 260,* 153-155. https://www.nature.com/articles/260153a0
9. Ayaki, M., et al. (2016). Protective effect of blue-light shield eyewear for adults against light pollution from self-luminous devices used at night. *Chronobiology International, 33*(1), 134-9. https://doi.org/10.3109/07420528.2015.1119158
10. Lin, J.B., et al. (2017). Short-Wavelength Light-Blocking Eyeglasses Attenuate Symptoms of Eye Fatigue. *Investigative Ophthalmology & Visual Science, 58*(1), 442-447. https://doi.org/10.1167/iovs.16-20663. PMID: 28118668.
11. Colombo, L., et al. (2017). Visual function improvement using photochromic and selective blue-violet light filtering spectacle lenses in patients affected by retinal diseases. *BMC Ophthalmology, 17*(1), 149. https://doi.org/10.1186/s12886-017-0545-9.
12. Bioregulatory Medicine Institute. (n.d.). *History - Edwin Dwight Babbitt, MD.* https://www.biologicalmedicineinstitute.com/edwin-dwight-babbitt
13. Sevinc, K. & Kingsley, O.K. (2014). The Effects of Color on the Moods of College Students. Sage Journals, 1-12. https://journals.sagepub.com/doi/10.1177/2158244014525423.

NOTES

14. The University of Arizona Health Sciences. (2020, September 9). *Shining a Green Light on a New Preventative Therapy for Migraine.* https://uahs.arizona.edu/tomorrow/shining-green-light-new-preventive-therapy-migraine
15. Pierce, Shanley. (2020, February 5). *Exposure to Green Light May Reduce Pain.* Texas Medical Center. https://www.tmc.edu/news/2020/02/exposure-to-green-light-may-reduce-pain/.
16. Ruggero, Cadossi, et al. (2020). "Pulsed Electromagnetic Field Stimulation of Bone Healin gand Joint Preservation: Cellular Mechanisms of Skeletal Response." Jounral of the American Academy of Orthopaedic Surgeons. May 2020. Vol 4, Issue 5. Web. Accessed Aug 20, 2021. https://journals.lww.com/jaaosglobal/Fulltext/2020/05000/Pulsed_Electromagnetic_Field_Stimulation_of_Bone.12.aspx.
17. Strauch, B., et al. (2009). Evidence-based use of pulsed electromagnetic field therapy in clinical plastic surgery. *Aesthetic Surgery Journal*, 29(2), 135-43. https://doi.org/10.1016/j.asj.2009.02.001
18. Larsen, E.R., et al. (2020). Transcranial pulsed electromagnetic fields for treatment-resistant depression: A multicenter 8-week single-arm cohort study. *European Psychiatry*, 63(1), e18. https://doi.org/10.1192/j.eurpsy.2020.3
19. Fiani, B., et al. (2021). Pulsed Electromagnetic Field Stimulators Efficacy for Noninvasive Bone Growth in Spine Surgery. *Journal of Korean Neurosurgical Society.* 64(4), 486–494. https://doi.org/10.3340/jkns.2020.0269
20. Goodwin, T.. (2006, January 1). *An Optimization of Pulsed Electro-Magnetic Fields Study.* NASA Johnson Space Center Houston, TX. https://ntrs.nasa.gov/citations/20070004785.
21. Lipton, B. (2008). *The Biology of Belief: Unleashing the Power of Consciousness, Matter & Miracles.* Hay House, Inc.
22. Sheldrake, R. (n.d). *Morphic Resonance and Morphic Fields - an Introduction.* Sheldrake.org. https://www.sheldrake.org/research/morphic-resonance/introduction

ACKNOWLEDGMENTS

I would like to thank Graceann Barrett who helped me write this book, Emily Daw in the editorial evaluation, Covered by Nicole in the cover design, and Jennifer Eaton in the book design and formatting.

CPSIA information can be obtained
at www.ICGtesting.com
Printed in the USA
JSHW081030020223
37134JS00005B/18